Touch the Earth

Jennifer Appleyard

*To Anne
with love
Jen*

HAYLOFT PUBLISHING LTD
KIRKBY STEPHEN

First published by Hayloft 2012

Hayloft Publishing Ltd, South Stainmore,
Kirkby Stephen, Cumbria, CA17 4DJ

tel: 017683 41568
email: books@hayloft.eu
web: www.hayloft.eu

ISBN 1 904524 72 9

A CIP catalogue record for this book is available from the British Library

Designed, printed and bound in the EU

Papers used by Hayloft are natural, recyclable products made from wood
grown in sustainable forest. The manufacturing processes conform to the
environmental regulations of the country of origin.

Cover photograph: Jane Dobinson, side saddle rider.

For David, Sally and Ann

CONTENTS

A man ought to do as well as a horse;
I wish all men did as well.

E. P. Rowe

PROLOGUE

Beaumont-Hamel Region, France, 1916

The young officer was close to death. He had slumped forwards in the saddle, his arms around the neck of the horse. Blood from a shrapnel wound in his chest dripped from the fingers of his left hand and mingled with the blood of the horse, which flowed from a large gaping hole in the animal's shoulder. The man's head was covered in congealed blood, black and red from a gash above his eyes, his matted hair indistinguishable from the mane upon which it lay.

The dampness of the late November afternoon had turned to drizzle which was soaking into the man's jacket and Sam Brown belt, and had saturated the horse's coat causing it to look dark brown, black even, emphasising the veins which stood out with effort.

Wearily the horse kept up a steady walk, though lame, dropping on its near fore, it held its head as high as exhaustion and loss of blood would permit, sensing the need to support the burden whose arms had already slackened. Had the officer been closer to consciousness he would have known the tremendous effort the animal was making in mustering the last of its strength.

Darkness began to fall and the battle sounds in the distance were lessening as a farm came into sight. Instinctively the horse made for it, stumbling up a tree lined rutted lane and into a muck strewn yard. Light spilled from a window silhouetting enquiring heads followed by a door swinging open and a couple of figures hurrying into the yard, pulling on their coats.

The elderly farmer reached the horse first, '*Mon Dieu*,' he breathed, his arms reaching to the injured rider, 'help me Monique.'

With difficulty they lowered the man from the saddle and half carried, half dragged him into the house. The woman tended him as best
she could, whilst her husband offered water to the horse, though it
showed little interest. Too far gone, the farmer thought with resignation. He harnessed their pony, backed it into the shafts of a trap, and
drove briskly to a field hospital some kilometres away, returning in
the darkness with a weary orderly who ministered to the officer's
wounds and requested he stay where he was until he could be moved.
By the time the farmer had returned to the farm, the dejected horse in
the yard could hardly stand, its head low to the ground. He led it into
a barn where he removed the army saddle and bridle and put on a
homemade hemp halter with which he tied the animal, then, wisped
its body down with a twist of straw and again proffered water.

The horse scarcely damped its mouth, more, the man felt, to oblige
him, for he was aware, even in its present condition, of undeniable
breeding. Holding the lamp higher the man examined the injury, tenderly feeling the large wound on the shoulder where the hide had been
ripped exposing muscle in which he could see metal glinting amongst
the clots of blood and torn flesh. He put a hand on the animal's neck
and spoke into the inert ears, 'I'll need to get that out before you'll
have a chance,' he told the horse and went back into the house for the
necessary aids.

A lifetime's experience of livestock gave him the courage he needed to tackle the injury. He explained quietly to the animal what he
was about to do, then with scrubbed hands he washed the wound with
water before dousing it with some of his precious brandy. The horse
flinched with the sting of it and made a deep guttural sound, but
accepted the ministrations, coping with the intricate removal of shrapnel, then the stretching and shaping of skin over the wound and homemade stitching with needle and thread dipped in the raw spirit.

With a wisdom before his time the man left a hole at the bottom
of the wound for drainage, remembering the words of his *grandpère*,
'Nature heals from the inside out, not the other way round as we
would have it.'

He began to wash some of the caked blood from the leg, continuing to talk softly, yet before he had finished the stallion collapsed to his knees and lay flat out on the straw bedding.

Inside the house the officer was barely conscious. The woman seated beside him wrung out cloths in cold water and lay them across his forehead. The bleeding had abated but the man was feverish and restless.

She turned to her husband as he entered the room, 'Will the horse live Jacques?'

'I've done all I can for it.'

'If it dies we'll have meat, we can feed our family and those of our neighbours.' She looked at him slyly, 'You'd have been best to kill it, put it out of its misery. God knows we could use it.'

From the bed there was a terrible cry as the man arched his back his eyes staring unseeing, 'No...'

PART ONE

UTOPIA

The blossom stars of sweetest scent
on boughs of Linden tree breeze bent,
yet for the briefest time they shine
fragrance of Heaven is freely thine.

Anonymous,
Old English

I

Through the darkness of the January evening, snowflakes the size of pennies were falling soundlessly. The slate roof of the red brick Georgian house was already covered as were those of three stable blocks to the east of it. The snow in the yards was deep, untrodden since the first flakes had fallen over an hour before. From the foaling block in the top yard nearest to the house, alien light spilled from the windows, cutting sharp edges through the snow, illuminating the density of its fall. In one of the foaling boxes the glow from numerous oil lamps was reflected on the faces of two men working with a mare struggling to give birth.

Watching, Elizabeth O'Malley Sullivan dug her nails into the palm of one hand whilst clutching the arm of her childhood companion, James Gretton, with the other. She found herself repeating her prayers to the Holy Mother, beseeching intercession for the foal to be born live, whilst not diverting her eyes from the efforts of the men labouring with the mare. She knew the presentation was normal, yet the birth was not progressing though the men had managed to secure foaling ropes onto the fetlocks of the foal which had been visible for some time.

John, her father, spoke through his efforts, 'Elizabeth, fetch more water and towels. James, go out and see if there's any sign of Angus.' He passed an arm across his forehead, wiping off the sweat which was running into his eyes as he said quietly to his companion, 'We've got a hell of a big foal here Tom, please God there's no complications to add to it.'

'It wouldn't be the first time,' Tom said, 'at least its head's not back, but we're going to have all on to get it safely.'

Out in the yard, Elizabeth, a bucket in each hand, hurried towards the tack room, whilst James made his way through the gates which had been fastened back some time before in anticipation of the vet's arrival. He peered down the village road, through the falling snow, hoping to see the lamps of the trap, yet there was nothing but swirling whiteness as far as he could see and the total stillness which accompanied it.

He turned back into the yard and joined Elizabeth in the tack room where she was filling buckets with warm water, their eyes met as he shook his head. She stared at him anxiously for a moment and then draped a couple of clean towels around her shoulders as James picked up a fresh tablet of soap and took the buckets from her and carried them back to the foaling box.

'No sign of the vet or the lad who went to fetch him,' James informed the men upon his return.

'We may have to fetch one or more of the grooms out then.' John looked to Tom, 'I'll soap her well and we'll have another try?'

'Right.'

The two youngsters took the taut rope from John and kept up the tension along with Tom.

Elizabeth held hard but knew that without James she could not have prevented the foal from slipping back, 'Hurry Papa,' she said, watching with anxious eyes as her father washed his hands for the umpteenth time and lathered soap around the vulva of the mare.

John dried his hands on a towel from his daughter's shoulders, then took over the rope and resumed the strong steady pulling. Muffled sounds came from the yard along with voices, but the men maintained their efforts. The mare grunted, her eyes rolling with pain and summoned her failing strength as the men worked with her.

To Elizabeth's enormous relief, the foal began to move forwards, slowly, and she felt the stirring of tears as she watched the miracle of the birth process.

'God, the size of it,' John gasped, as the shoulders were eased out and the delivery was held up by the foal's hips, the young animal hanging by them.

'Take its weight Tom, whilst I work on its quarters,' John said hoarsely, as the door of the loose box opened and Angus McLoughlin strode in. Without a word, the vet grabbed a towel from Elizabeth and helped Tom support the slippery body, whilst John's strong fingers manipulated the hips out. Then, with a rush of fluids, the foal slid from the mare, its birth sac half around it.

Tom bent over the foal and cleaned out its mouth and nostrils, wiping the airways with a towel. The foal spluttered out the rest as Tom put a hand between its back legs.

'A colt.'

John nodded.

Angus checked the mare. 'You've done well,' he said succinctly, 'you haven't torn her.'

'Thank God for a safe delivery,' John spoke the words which generations of O'Malley's had said over live births. The group nodded their responses as the mare turned to her foal.

'Sorry Angus, to fetch you out on such a night,' John spoke over his shoulder whilst washing his hands and arms.

'I wish all my foalings were so easy,' Angus said dourly, 'all I did was open the door.'

'And help me support the foal,' Tom said seriously, 'I've seen hanging like that damage their lungs.'

'Aye, you're right Tom, they can't hang for long.'

John dried himself and pulled on his jersey, 'Unless I'm much mistaken, this is the colt we've been hoping for. The tenacity of Bridgitte's line with the confirmation and colour of his sire, Bladhaire.' He stood back and studied the foal, 'It's my guess he'll be an even brighter chestnut than Bladhaire. Mark my words, he'll be as red as the heads on the Galway coast. Will you look at him?'

He inclined his head, though the assembly needed no urging for they hadn't taken their eyes off the colt since he had dropped into the world.

'You'll be leaving him entire then?' Angus asked.

'Too true Angus. He'll be a stallion in a million.'

✤ ✤ ✤

After Bridgitte had been given warm water to drink and a bran mash dampened with porter, John and Tom transferred the lamps into the passageway where they threw flickering shadows through the bars above the wooden partitions and left the twelve-year-olds to keep watch.

The three men made for the house and John's office, to wet the foal's head and air their usual differences of the merits of Irish versus Scotch whisky.

Elizabeth and James perched themselves high on a pile of straw in the neighbouring stall, chins resting on arms laid alongside the top of the loose box and watched as the mare nickered softly to her foal whilst she cleaned it with her tongue, content now the birth struggle was over. They watched the foal put every ounce of his developing strength into his attempts to get up and eventually wobbling towards his dam, splaying his long legs whilst bending his head to nuzzle her, seeking a teat and the nourishment which would grow him into John's prediction.

Elizabeth nudged James as the foal began to suck strongly, he returned the pressure and she felt the shared relief as their elbows remained in contact. She thought of the many times herself and James had helped with foals and foalings and was proud that she had inherited 'a feel for mares.' The unselfconscious weight of James' arm against hers reminded her that he too had this gift, having grown up as Tom's own child, shadowing him and absorbing all that Tom taught him. Elizabeth felt the warmth of growing self confidence steal over her, knowing that both she and James could be relied on to carry out most of the tasks in the day to day running of a large stud farm and were encouraged to do so.

The snow had ceased to fall when after an hour or so the three men returned and the lad had brought the pony and trap into the yard for the vet's return.

Tom listened intently to Elizabeth and James' whispered report.

'He's done well then after a tiring birth, but for all he's a strong colt, I always rest easier when they've started sucking. Now let's be having the two of you, it's late and long past your bedtime.' He smiled indulgently as the youngsters slid down from the straw.

'Will..?'

'You know I will,' Tom replied to Elizabeth, anticipating her question. 'Don't I always have a look in during the first night or two?'

Elizabeth nodded, yawning through a smile, 'Always. Good night then.' She made her way through the snow, across the yard, to the postern door of the house.

✄ ✄ ✄

John had left a lamp burning in the mud room, where Elizabeth shed her breeches, boots and thick jersey, scrubbed her hands and pulled on clean house clothes. After turning out the lantern she hurried to the family sitting room, adjusting her pace as she opened the door, in deference to her mother's frail health.

John and Mary were sitting each side of a dying fire in the light thrown by the tall chimneys of crystal oil lamps, behind which red brocade curtains were drawn against the January night. Elizabeth felt the familiar comfort within the room envelop her.

John took his feet off a footstool and offered it to her. She kissed her mother's forehead before sinking down onto the stool which she pulled nearer to the hearth, stretching out her hands towards the remaining embers.

Mary's cheeks dimpled at Elizabeth's shining eyes and ready smile. 'Well my dear, I don't have to ask after the new foal, I can tell by the look of you that he's fine.'

Elizabeth gazed up at Mary's tranquil face, 'We had a job with him Mama, we could have lost him, but Papa and Tom were wonderful.' She reached for her father's hand and kissed the palm. 'Papa thinks that this colt has it all. Just think, we can use him on many of the mares not related to him or his line. I'm going to get the stud books out and James and I can begin to compile a list.'

'Good Lord,' John interrupted, 'the creature's barely arrived and you're planning years ahead.' He laughed loudly, crossing the room to a mahogany card table and hovered over a silver tray, 'Night-cap anyone?'

Mary shook her head.

'Let's, Mama. A ginger beer to toast the colt?'

John opened two stone bottles and poured ginger beer, then helped himself to a generous measure of Jameson whiskey. He handed Mary and Elizabeth their drinks then raised his glass, 'To... whatever his name is.' He closed his eyes and thought for a moment, then his face broke into the smile that Elizabeth loved, '*Rua,* Irish for red,' then. 'Tell me Elizabeth, what's King in the Irish?'

Elizabeth screwed up her face in concentration, '*Ri,* Papa, with the *shina fada* above the i, so it's pronounced Ree.'

Mary looked at Elizabeth in feigned amazement, 'You have been working at Papa's beloved Irish after all. There is more to life than horses then?'

'*Ri Rua*, the noun before the adjective in Irish, so Red King. How about that for his name?' John asked.

Elizabeth nodded well pleased with her father's choice, 'Perfect Papa,' she said touching her glass to those of her parents in turn. 'To Ri Rua,' she said.

৯৫ ৯৫ ৯৫

Later, after Mary and Elizabeth had gone to their beds, John returned to the office. He rolled back the top of the desk taking out his files, where he meticulously recorded the birth of the colt before leaning back in the swivel chair, well content with the evening's business. He looked up above his desk to the large portrait of his grandfather Gerard, mounted on his favourite hunter, Bruth, a powerful grey. It might well be a picture of himself, John thought, as he had many times before. The same medium height, strong build, and dark hair.

What a character Gerard must have been, driven by the poverty of his family to leave his native Ireland and seek work in England to support them. His sheer physical effort, often to exhaustion, easing their lot and eventually securing for himself the modest holding in Derbyshire where the O'Malley Stud still grazed their young stock.

John stared into Gerard's blue eyes, so like his own, and thought of the standing Gerard had earned as a reputable dealer and breeder of hunters. Amongst his associates was Percival, then Squire of Oakley, a man whose infamy had followed him down through the years as a drinker and a rake. A card game - all that Gerard had against the Oakley farm he had recently rented, now the O'Malley stud. John still found the story almost unbelievable. Won by a turn of the cards. Gerard he felt, would be well pleased with the dedication of his descendants and of the international reputation the O'Malley Stud had gained in the years which had followed.

The increasing, troubled, rumblings across Europe seemed far away from Oakley and all that John held precious there.

II

The past four and a half years had brought few changes to Oakley, for all the clock on the ancient parish church had tolled the hours of over sixteen hundred days and nights.

Elizabeth felt that heaven could be no better than riding Rua as she schooled him in the paddock in front of the house. His tremendous controlled strength took her breath away as did his response to her aids, whilst she walked, trotted and cantered him in circles and figure eights, her legs in close contact with his sides, the subtle changes in her body weight conveying to him more clearly than words what she expected of him. She felt exhilarated and totally at one with the horse.

John leant on the gate of the paddock and watched his daughter ride whilst he awaited buyers from Holland. God, he was proud of her, what a character she was, so like his mother Grainnie and not only in looks either, he decided, particularly now she was older, but in her ability to communicate with horses, a gift he had known and admired in his mother.

'By all the Saints, she can ride,' a voice broke quietly into John's thoughts as Tom joined him at the gate.

'She can too, I was just thinking how like her grandmother she gets.' Tom nodded, his eyes on Elizabeth.

John stared beyond the paddock to the tidy railed off fields where brood mares and their foals grazed.

'I remember my mother the last time I saw her,' he said quietly, 'she was so vital and alive, mounted side saddle on a handsome black gelding, navy habit, white stock, top hat with a tight veil around her beautiful face, eyes as blue as the summer sky.'

He rubbed his hand across his forehead, 'She blew a kiss to me at an upstairs window. I'd been ill and was confined to the house you see. Then they were gone, she and a groom riding her second horse. It had been early in the season, an outing to give the horse some experience in the field as much as anything, a normal day in our lives.'

'Aye.'

'The day seemed interminable. I'd tried to catch up with my studies, but couldn't concentrate on them. Then I heard the clatter of hooves on the gravel and the sound of voices. I looked down from the window, the groom was riding the second horse and had led the black home. The late squire and his huntsman were in the yard, their faces drained of colour, they broke the news to my father that my mother was dead. The horse had come down jumping a wall and she had hit her head on a loose stone as the two fell to the ground. They said it was instantaneous.'

'Grievous,' Tom's kindly weathered face creased in sympathy for the man who was both his employer and his friend. Though he had always been aware of the tragic hunting accident which had robbed John of his mother, he had never heard John speak of it in detail. He took off his cap and smoothed back his greying dark hair before replacing it.

The two men stood together in silence for a while. Tom turned his attention back to Elizabeth and was as poignantly moved as John by her unity with the horse.

'There's credit due to Elizabeth, and James too for what they've done with that horse,' he finally commented.

John returned his gaze to his daughter. 'Yes, that's for sure, I think we were wise to let them work so closely with him, for all it worried us, him being an entire.'

'Aye, fortunately he's got the most amiable temperament I've known in a stallion. Add his looks and intelligence to that...'

'Yes, he really is something,' John agreed.

They were interrupted by the approach of James.

'The Dutch buyers are here Mr. O'Malley.'

'Thank you James,' John turned to Tom. 'Right Tom, let's go and see what business we can do.'

Elizabeth acknowledged the departure of her father and Tom with a nod, then urged the stallion to lengthen his stride into an extended trot. She glanced at James from the corner of her eye and smiled as he raised his thumbs. Then she walked the horse around for a while before pulling him in at the gate and stroking his neck, conscious of his powerful presence combined with the good manners of which her father was so insistent. No one was more aware than she, that horses bearing the O'Malley prefix were expected to do the stud the credit for which their name had become synonymous.

James took the horse from her and as they settled Rua in his box they discussed him enthusiastically.

'How about that trot then? Doesn't he just float?'

James nodded as he flicked a brush across the horse's back, 'Perfect. I reckon he's the best horse I've ever ridden. Who was it who quoted, '*riding the west wind*?' and there's nothing he won't try, he's got one hell of a jump.'

'He's brilliant,' Elizabeth laid her head on the horse's shoulder, 'I know at first that Papa was not overjoyed at him being ridden so much, but he finally agrees that a well schooled entire has it all.' She stroked the silky neck and lowered her voice conspiringly, 'Did you know that the elders have actually suggested that I school him more in a side saddle? What do you think of that?' She smiled as she used the title they frequently gave to John and Tom in their absence.

'Essential if you're hunting him this season. Well as you ride astride, it wouldn't do out hunting.' James tutted reproachfully and grinned, his teeth shining white in the semi-gloom of the stable.

Elizabeth lowered her eyes in mock submission, 'Oh, I wouldn't dream of riding astride to hounds, I don't much care myself but I'd be an embarrassment to my parents and as for our dear master, I fear it would bring on his apoplexy.' She pulled a face before returning his grin.

James finished brushing the glossy coat and settled the dust sheet over the horse's back. Automatically she passed him the surcingle, their hands meeting under the horse's belly.

'I wish it would bring on apoplexy to his son, I can't stand Robert Oakley,' James buckled the roller, adding, 'I know you've always mixed with him and his sisters but the less I see of him the better. He's a prig.'

'He's not so bad, just self opinionated.'

James looked hard at her over Rua's back, 'I've never liked to think of you being around him, not ever. There's something about him. I can't really explain. Something sinister, and the way he treats people...' James hesitated for a moment. 'You must always be wary of him Beth, I think...' He tightened his lips and Elizabeth watching him, felt he was beginning to regret broaching the subject. It did not, she found, prevent him from finishing what he had intended to say. 'I think he's capable of doing people harm.'

An uncomfortable silence fell between them, Elizabeth studied the horse's ears, now still, which had previously been moving around following their voices. 'You can't mean that. Why do you say it?'

'It's a feeling I've got about him. I've always had it.'

She scrutinised his face, 'It's not like you to be fanciful James, whatever's come over you?'

He shrugged and letting the horse free, followed her out and disappeared into the tack room.

❧ ❧ ❧

Elizabeth wandered off down the orchard and unhampered by skirts, for she was still wearing breeches, boots and a well worn shirt, climbed the stile and walked into the mowing grass. She knew her father would be extremely displeased by this sacrilege but dismissed the knowledge impatiently, for she felt unsettled and oddly disturbed. As though the action would free her from such elusive emotions, she unloosed her hair, shook it out and ran into the full sun of the June afternoon throwing herself down into the fragrant herbage. The feeling of disquiet however, remained as she mulled over what James had said. Robert Oakley... she closed her eyes, seeing his narrow, pale face as he patronised his sisters and her, too, on occasions, and she shuddered involuntarily.

A bee noisily working clover heads close by failed to distract her endeavours to understand James' foreboding. His face replaced that of Robert in her mind, his regular, tanned features, the dimple in his chin, one so familiar in her life. She thought of his capable nature and ability with horses, the legacy of Tom's upbringing. Absently she pulled up a blade of rye grass and chewed on its sweet stalk. It had been inevitable, she realised, that she and James would grow up so in tune for they had always been inseparable, bonded by their mutual passion for horses. Elizabeth never failed to appreciate the freedom her father gave her in an age when her contemporaries were discouraged from putting as much as a toe out of line.

She knew her mother had been won over to her father's way of raising her by John's proud talk of his own mother, whose reputation as a fearless rider was still a legend across three counties. Had Elizabeth but known, her thoughts ran along similar lines to those of her father less than an hour before. Grainnie O'Malley Sullivan, her grandmother, claimed her family could be traced back to Grace O'Malley, more often remembered around the west coast of Ireland as Granuaile, legendary leader of the O'Malley clan in the 1500s. Elizabeth knew the story by heart from her father's repeated tales of this indomitable ancestor who had not been afraid to tackle the English Queen regarding the atrocities perpetrated by the Crown Administrator upon her sons and their followers. Elizabeth remembered asking as a young child, 'Is it for the Queen that I was so named?'

Her father had expostulated, 'Indeed child it was not. You are named for the Holy Cousin of the Blessed Virgin, Elizabeth, mother of the Baptist no less.' She recalled even now, so long afterwards how he had shaken his head most emphatically, 'The English Queen indeed.'

Elizabeth was so immersed in her thoughts that when the sun was shielded from her closed eyelids she had to recall her whereabouts for a moment. She opened her eyes as James sat down in the long grass beside her.

'I thought I saw you coming here, just what do you think you're doing in one of the hay fields?' His shock was evident to her.

'What are you?' Elizabeth retorted more sharply than she had intended.

James didn't answer, he looked up, his eyes following the flight of a lark as it climbed almost out of sight, its song becoming more faint, then roughly combed his fingers through his untidy sun bleached hair and rolled onto his stomach. He looked at her intently. Elizabeth met his gaze. The pupils of his eyes, she saw, were huge, the grey surrounds hardly visible. For the first time she noticed he shaved, for his skin was smooth where not long since it had been heavy down and she felt her face flushing as the realisation of how much he had altered without her noticing, dawned upon her. His voice, she recalled, had become different for some time. She studied the line of his jaw, the sideburns by his ears and her senses reeled as she awoke to the sheer masculinity of him.

He didn't take his eyes from hers and instinctively she knew that he was finding in her a person unknown to him also, one whose company he had taken for granted in the same way that she herself had done. Elizabeth felt her legs weaken and her abdomen twist strangely as his close proximity seemed to stifle her breathing and she was overwhelmed by a painful embarrassment which she would never have expected to feel in his company. James reached out a hand and stroked back a tendril of dark hair from her forehead. His fingers seemed to hold an electric current which sparked against the side of her face whilst she continued to look up at him.

How long they gazed at each other as they lay in the forbidden mowing grass Elizabeth could never really remember, only that from then on they were both hesitant of any physical contact as they continued to work together in stilted and tangible awareness. Elizabeth had been right in her assumption that James had also experienced a startling awakening on that early June afternoon.

For one who rose so early James had slept very little since. In the cottage to the rear of the top yard, he lay awake night after night. The moon, filtering through the cotton curtains cast the shape of the iron bedstead in shadow onto the floor by his side. Endlessly he recalled those moments. Endlessly he re-lived standing beside Elizabeth as she lay in the hayfield, the neck of her shirt open, the swell of her young breasts just visible, her dark hair loose and tangled around her head, her lips full and tender as she had spoken. Again he felt the cool grass beneath him as he had lain on his stomach beside her, crushing the churning in his abdomen, feeling for her a desire which had sprung into life in those moments. The sensation of losing himself in her eyes, so blue, so dark... he had known then as now, without a shadow of doubt, that things would never be the same between them again.

For all her father employed his uncle and now himself, James realised that John O'Malley Sullivan was a unique man, one with no patience with class or position, judging every man on his merits. As a consequence James knew, due to his inseparability with Elizabeth, he had in the past grown as close to her as a brother, one who had taken care of her, restrained her impulsive nature from childhood, saved her from often reckless ventures. He remembered, how only a year or two ago, he had pulled her out of the old moat when she had got into difficulties rescuing a hen and he had managed to get her undetected into the tack room where he had stirred up the fire, helped her undress and rubbed her down with stable cloths, thinking no more about it than drying off a horse. This memory at least caused him to smile as he saw again the skinny little girl shivering in the horse blanket he had wrapped around her whilst she waited for her clothes to dry and contrary to her nature, listened to his admonishment.

How would he cope with her in that predicament now, he asked himself as his body stirred unbidden and shame challenged it. So many memories, for although they were of an age, he had, as far back as he could remember, felt the need to protect her, which, seemed in his confusion, contradictory to the instincts which had been released in him so short a time ago.

III

Saxon Brown clattered into the top yard of the O'Malley stables on his big grey gelding Dolomite, expertly closing the side gate behind him. A few of the lads who came in daily from the village put their heads over the half doors.

'Beth,' he boomed leaning forwards in the saddle, then receiving no response, dismounted and offered his reins to a lad who had come out. He ran up the curving brick steps to the house and thumped the door with his crop. Elizabeth's head appeared at an upstairs window, 'Good morning Saxon, sorry I'm not ready, I've been having a fitting for the new gown I'll be wearing at the summer ball.'

'Never mind all that folderol Beth. It's too good a morning, hurry down and let's get off riding before the sun's any higher.'

Within minutes Elizabeth appeared in the yard dressed in her everyday habit, black skirt covering breeches and boots, anticipating the promise of a hot day by wearing a white linen shirt, her hair coiled at her neck. She fondled the muzzle of Dolomite as she passed, nodding to the lad who was holding him and made for her mare Minette. Tom was just finishing grooming her whilst Saxon leaned on the manger talking to him.

'Morning Tom, looks a though it's going to be a scorcher.'

'Aye it does that Elizabeth. She's ready for you.'

Elizabeth smiled and helped him tack up the mare, then Tom led her out to the stone steps in the corner of the yard, where Elizabeth mounted side saddle, whilst Tom checked the balancing girth. She arranged her skirt, gathered up the reins and waited for Saxon to mount. The grey pranced once he was mounted attempting half rears in his eagerness to be off. Tom watching, raised his eyebrows to Elizabeth who had automatically glanced at him during the horse's performance.

'Don't let him get away with bad manners Saxon,' she called to him.

Saxon laughed, 'He's alright, just a show off like me, anxious to be away with two beautiful females.'

Elizabeth shook her head and raising a hand to Tom at the gate preceded Saxon out of the yard. The village main street with its straggling cottages, gave way to a bridle path lined by giant beech trees, their small pleated leaves rustling lazily overhead.

They rode close, Elizabeth on Saxon's nearside to prevent her lower leg from being caught by his stirrup iron. She was completely at ease in his company for they had enjoyed an easy friendship from childhood. The Browns were their nearest neighbours, farming the land west of the stud. Elizabeth shared their tutor and would do until Saxon followed his elder brother Edward, to Durham University. Regularly she and Saxon would hack over to local meets together, for his family raced their hunters in the annual point to points and needed to be seen out with hounds on enough occasions to qualify.

Without suggestion or comment they made for their favourite ride, Lamcote hills, crossing two bridges on the bridle road, one over the railway, the other spanning the dark canal. Ahead of them Elizabeth could see the comfortable bulk of a local farmer, with his pony and trap. She guessed he was off to Nottingham Market, his large brood of children ran along the hedgeside shouting their goodbyes, then returned their attention to a fat pony they had been trying to catch. The group paused for long enough to wave to Elizabeth and Saxon then continued their endeavours with the reluctant animal.

Elizabeth watched them with amusement as she and Saxon rode by, until the hills, which offered the best gallop around, were upon them. Catching Saxon's eye and with a shout of 'Now,' she spurred the mare, pressing her hard up the first of the three hills. With a perfectly balanced seat, she leaned forwards into the wind rush, sensing sooner than hearing Dolomite thundering up behind her. The gelding pounded the ground and drew alongside her. The mare felt to Elizabeth as though she was stroking the turf from under her. More lightly built than the gelding, Elizabeth knew that Minette could fly over short distances. They raced neck and neck down the first hill, the second rose and fell, one more to go. Elizabeth pushed the mare into the last rise and hurtled down the other side, then together they galloped out into open country, breathless and exhilarated. The mare had won, but only just, for Elizabeth knew that the gelding had been settling into the powerful stride which was already the making of him.

Saxon grinned, blue eyes streaming, his tawny hair sticking up like a lion's mane. Elizabeth leaned forward and patted the mare's neck as they slowed down into walking pace, side by side.

'No matter where we give the horses a good pipe opener, there's nowhere to beat the hills.'

'Yes, I get damn nearly as much fun out of it here as I do racing, especially with you Beth, by God you can ride and it's more than my life's worth to say 'for a girl'.' He cast a glance at her, seeing to his amusement that she avoided his eyes, her cheeks flushed with more than exertion.

Elizabeth spoke as though she hadn't heard him, 'Will Edward be home in time for the ball, Saxon?'

'I don't think he'd miss it for the world. He's rather fond of Sarah Oakley you know.'

'Really, but then I suppose they've always been good friends. Haven't we all over the years.'

'It's becoming a bit more than that from what I can make out. They're writing to each other.'

Elizabeth raised her eyebrows, 'Goodness, I suppose that's quite romantic.'

Saxon grimaced, 'I'd sooner ride this fellow in a point to point than get involved with any of that.' He slapped the horse's shoulder to emphasise his preference.

'When do you think people normally become interested in romance then Saxon?'

He looked at her sideways an amused smile playing about his mouth, 'Oh, I should think in your twenties, quite old, wouldn't you?'

'You haven't anyone particular you're hoping to see at the ball then?'

'Good Lord no. I'll dance with you, Beth, you've never minded my treading on your toes, rotten dancer, always was.'

Elizabeth pulled a face at him, 'Don't I know it. How many times have I suffered bruised feet and laddered silk stockings as the result of your clodhopping attempts at dancing? You don't seem to improve. I'm not so sure I can stand it again, you might have to find another partner, someone blissfully unaware of your dancing skills, or rather lack of them.'

He roared with laughter and wiped his eyes with the back of his hand, 'You don't mean that. You're a pal, one of my best pals in fact, I think I'll save myself for you, could do a lot worse than you Beth.'

Elizabeth laughed despite herself, 'Don't ever change Saxon, I wouldn't really like you to.' She was quiet for a few moments, then, 'Have you noticed how people change? You know like Edward and Sarah for instance, friends all their lives then suddenly something else? A completely different relationship, isn't it strange? How do you think they feel about the change? It seems almost unbelievable how our feelings for people can become something quite different.'

He looked directly at her, as if willing himself to make sense of what she was trying to say, knowing that she was stumbling somehow and yet feeling hopelessly inadequate to deal with it.

⚜ ⚜ ⚜

They fell silent for a while as they rode on across the fields towards Lowerton village, passing the Admiral Nelson Inn and cluster of cottages around the church.

Saxon inclined his head in the direction of Lowerton Hall and leaned towards Elizabeth conspiringly, 'Talking of relationships, no need to wonder whom our friend Robert will be favouring at the ball. He'll be under orders to be charm itself to Miss Victoria Burdette, you mark my words.'

Elizabeth stared at him, 'Well now that's interesting,' she nodded perspicaciously. 'You probably have something there. Land marries land in their circles especially when parts of it are adjacent.'

'Your land borders that of the Oakleys you know, he might well transfer his attentions in your direction.'

Elizabeth looked at him sharply and caught him grinning, she laughed, 'Absolute rubbish Saxon, and you know it, our land is fractional compared to the Lowerton estate.'

He was serious for a moment, 'All I wish for you Beth, is your happiness.'

'Saxon, you're a dear, there aren't many people like you or your family, that's why I count you amongst my very best friends, therefore as a special concession I shall dance with you on Saturday evening and bear the pain stoically.'

'You're a sport,' he grinned wryly, 'for a girl!'

She drew her eyebrows together in a mock scowl and set Minette into a canter, scattering the pollen from meadowsweet which lined the grass verge as they headed in the direction of Oakley.

The week fled. John was in Ireland negotiating sales with his Sullivan cousins, whilst Elizabeth and James were working with the young stock under the watchful eye of Tom. They rode out each day, exercising the youngsters, encouraging their confidence in the sights and sounds met on the roads out of the village en route to Nottingham. They showed the young horses the nearest railway station at Kelingleigh, familiarising them with the goods yard and livestock wagons which they used frequently.

It was towards the end of the week whilst out riding exercise with James, that Elizabeth brought up the subject of the ball. As soon as she had uttered the words she felt she could have bitten her tongue for she was still aware that the atmosphere between them was not as it had been. Her words were met by a stony silence as she contemplated her foolishness.

Then, 'Dancing with Robert Oakley I suppose?'

'Of course not James, he'll hardly notice me. I usually dance with

Saxon Brown, haven't you noticed I limp for a week afterwards, he's absolutely hopeless, but preferable by far to Robert.'

James bit his lip and turned his head, staring across the fields apparently absorbed in watching figures haymaking in the distance.

'James, please stop this. I've no interest in Robert Oakley. He's just, well, always been there I suppose, but so have his sisters, like Saxon and his brother.'

'Saxon's alright,' James retorted, 'I've always liked him, he's down to earth, not like some.'

'It might interest you to know, since Robert Oakley seems to be an obsession with you lately, that I've heard from a reliable source the Oakleys' have set their sights on Victoria Burdette for him, so what have you to make of that?'

'Victoria Burdette? Compared to you she's insignificant.'

'Don't say that. I've always found Victoria to be a most pleasant, gentle person and after all it's what someone is like inside that matters.'

He laughed mirthlessly, 'Well no one in their right mind would always call you pleasant and gentle and I should know, I've seen you in some right old tantrums Miss Elizabeth.'

'Oh have you, well you're going out of your way to cause another one now. I can't think what's got into you. Do you know I've always admired your level headedness. I can't remember a time when you haven't been there for me, not just as a friend, but a cornerstone of safety and... normalness and all the things I most value. Why have you changed?' The insecurity she had been trying to communicate to Saxon washed over her, leaving her feeling vulnerable and confused.

'Because I'm damned if I'll see you hurt, anyone but you could see what his type is. God knows he was a spoilt child and now as a result, he's the kind of man who will have his own way at all costs. Whatever he wants, he gets. You're not a child anymore Beth and he'll be more than aware of that.'

Elizabeth felt frustration turning to anger, 'Why are you keeping on about him. Once and for all, I've no interest whatsoever in Robert

Oakley and I can assure you that he would never have an interest in me because of my faith. You know as well as I do that even in this day and age Catholics are put outside much of society. In any event, I would never compromise my faith. You're Catholic yourself, would you?'

'No, I wouldn't but there's plenty of people who have, look at Queen Mary for a start, she soon turned her back on her Catholic faith for the English crown. They say that her father of Teck died of a broken heart because of it.'

'I didn't know that,' Elizabeth said slowly, 'how awful.' Then raised her voice to him, 'Whatever do you really think of me? I'm beginning to wonder if I know you at all James, or else you've changed from the person I have known.' Her forehead creased as she looked across at him, 'I think you've changed towards me, I don't think you care a fig for me anymore.'

He looked at her incredulously, 'How can you say that, just how can you?'

Elizabeth heard the bitter hurt in his voice and felt that the words between them were escalating out of control, it all seemed so unnecessary to her. She reached for his hand on the reins, 'James, I should never have said that, after all you've been like a brother to me.'

James clutched her hand against his thigh, 'I'd kill anyone who hurt you, make no mistake about that Beth.' His voice she noticed was low and hoarse and his grey eyes met hers with a fierce intensity that she found almost frightening.

IV

July, 1914

Robert Oakley posed before the cheval mirror in his dressing room. Well bred, handsome devil, he concluded, smiling to himself as his pale blue eyes surveyed his reflection, taking in the elegant height, fine boned face and aquiline nose. His tailor, Robert considered, had made a splendid job of the new tail coat in lightweight wool especially sent down from Preston's mill in Bolton. At his neck a crisp white shirt and white bow tie accentuated the well rehearsed lift of his head, quite Byronesque, Robert smiled, gratified by the comparison. Then wandering into his bedroom he crossed to one of the high sash windows and scanned the parkland with its carriage road, along which many of their guests would be travelling. The thought prompted him to pull out a gold hunter watch from the pocket of his white waistcoat and glance at the time. Join his father for a drink, he decided, fortify himself for the onslaught and ingratiating attention he must pay to Miss Victoria Burdette in compliance with filial obedience.

Squire Ralph Oakley with his slight, faded but pretty wife, Lenora and their younger daughter Hannah, were already in the library when Robert entered. They stood by the windows which also afforded a view of the carriage road in order to see the arrival of their guests.

'Robert dear, you look so elegant,' Lenora met him and linking her arm through his, tilted her head in her husband's direction inviting a similar response.

'Hum, must say I agree with your mother, very smart, nice piece of cloth from Walter Preston, what? Drink?' He nodded to a footman standing to attention by the double doors.

Robert scrutinised his sister, 'Couldn't you have done something with your hair Hannah? For God's sake look at her.'

Hannah's shoulders drooped visibly, causing her white Nottingham lace gown to sag. With a nervous glance at her brother, she twisted a handkerchief into knots and then stared miserably at the ground.

Lenora smiled indulgently, 'Robert dear, don't be unkind to your sister. I had my own maid dress Hannah's hair, I positively scrimped on the time she spent with me so that the child could benefit. Hannah has very difficult hair, I'm sure Esther has done her best with it, she's so clever.' She patted her own impeccable coiffure.

Robert cast a withering look at his sister, it seemed to him that more sprouts of her mousy hair had escaped from the pins than were restrained by them. He closed his eyes against the sight and turned his attention to his father who held up his drink.

'Here's to an enjoyable evening.' The family raised their glasses, joining his toast.

'Where's Sarah?' Robert queried, his forehead creasing. 'Really I seem to have the most tiresome sisters.'

Hannah stopped twisting the handkerchief and looked up, her face becoming animated. 'She's watching out of the windows for Edward Brown to arrive, isn't it exciting, I think they're falling in love.' She giggled and resumed her study of the floor.

'Hush child,' Lenora tutted as Ralph pushed his face close to Hannah's.

'What's that she's saying? Edward Brown?'

Lenora nodded, 'Yes dear, she seems to be very taken with him.'

'Good God,' Ralph nodded to the footman for more whisky. 'Well I suppose he's got more upstairs than that wild younger brother, the one who rides in the point to points.' He tapped the side of his head. 'Stark raving mad that one and have you seen him on the dance floor, like an elephant don't you know?' He indicated to the footman in Robert's direction, 'Fill us both up while you're at it, if we've got an evening ahead entertaining the county and half the neighbouring one, might as well brace ourselves, eh Robert, brace ourselves.' He laughed with little humour.

The tapping of shoes could be heard across the hall tiles and with a rustle of silk Sarah burst into the room. 'The Brown's carriage is half way up the hill. I've seen it from the west wing, they'll be coming round the drive any moment now, come along all of you, be ready to meet them as they arrive.' She bit her lips and pinched her cheeks frantically, then picked up her skirts and ran from the room with the same urgency that she had entered it.

'Sarah,' her mother called after her. 'Compose yourself, whatever will Mr and Mrs Brown think of you.' She relinquished Robert's arm and taking that of her husband went forth to greet the first of their guests.

In the middle yard of the O'Malley Stud, two of the grooms led out the team of bays whilst a stable lad opened the high doors of the coach house and the horses were backed into the family carriage. When the turnout met with the groom's criteria, the carriage was driven round to the front of the house and the lad was sent to knock on the door. John answered and smiling genially, ushered Mary and Elizabeth down the steps and onto the gravel where he assisted them into the carriage.

✀ ✀ ✀

From a gap made by a slipped tile in the loft of the top yard, James watched Elizabeth leave for the ball. He caught his breath at her loveliness. Her hair, he saw, was fastened in a twist at her neck with beads sparkling amongst it and her face was radiant, blue eyes shining, dark lashes sweeping her flushed cheeks. James, though not remotely interested in fashion, realised that the gown she wore was something quite special. He could only appreciate that it was of a filmy fabric the exact blue of her eyes and clung provocatively to her slender figure.

Then she was gone, the carriage doors closed and the horses

hooves crunching on the gravel as the family were driven away in the direction of Oakley Hall. James wrestled miserably with his thoughts. How had she altered this much and why had he been so unaware of it until recently? Why? He asked himself, had he been so churlish to her lately. What lasting damage had he done to their relationship? He remained in the loft for some time after Elizabeth had left, suffering a turmoil of self recrimination which he felt was almost more than he could bear. Added to this was the recurring foreboding that somehow Robert Oakley represented a threat to Elizabeth.

❧ ❧ ❧

The five piece orchestra was already playing from the gallery as John, Mary and Elizabeth entered the salon. They were warmly greeted by Ralph and Lenora, whose regard for them was apparent, the squire having infinite admiration for the O'Malley reputation and his wife charmed by Mary's graciousness and the fortitude with which she bore her failing health.

Ralph indicated to a huge silver punch bowl dominating a double pedestal table by the door. Tomkins, the Oakley's butler attended to them personally.

'Whisky for us eh John? Be damned to this pap.' He avoided his wife's eye. 'We'll settle down in the library later for some serious drinking, after supper when the dancing warms up, can't be doing with dancing myself.'

John laughed, 'More likely gout, you old fraud.'

'Never could keep much from you, too sharp by half,' Ralph remonstrated, smiling wryly.

Elizabeth had barely raised the drink to her lips when she received a hearty slap on the back which shot the contents of her glass across the floor. She turned to see Saxon hovering over her pulling a large handkerchief out of his pocket and brandishing it in her direction, 'Sorry Beth, has it spoil your gown?'

Elizabeth shook her head, 'No, by a miracle.' She was relieved of the empty glass by Tomkins who refilled it before directing a footman to mop up the spillage.

Ralph rolled his eyes to the O'Malleys' as Saxon continued, changing his weight from one foot to the other. 'I am a clumsy devil, my mother says I'm not fit to be inside as there's nowhere big enough to contain me and that I'm better suited to the great outdoors.'

He looked so contrite that Elizabeth's good humour was restored, 'Then maybe we'd be better outside for a while, can you be trusted to carry the drinks without further incident?'

'I'll make every effort.'

Alternate long sash windows opened up from floor level and many of the guests were already wandering around the lawns and gardens for although the sun was sinking, the July evening was warm and balmy. The Squire and his lady were upholding the time honoured tradition of throwing the summer ball between hay and harvest by the end of which they would provide a harvest supper for their farm workers and those on the estate's tenanted farms.

Elizabeth and Saxon walked slowly side by side across the lawn to the front of the hall where he gallantly wiped an ornamental bench with his handkerchief and handed over her glass with exaggerated care.

'You're overdoing it now.'

'Nothing's too good for you Beth,' he smiled his wide smile and Elizabeth looking up at him felt the corners of her mouth lifting, her expression reflecting his unfailing cheerfulness.

Elizabeth looked at the hall, moved as always by the sheer age of the parts where the great corner stones had been taken from the same quarry as those of the medieval church close by. 'Isn't the hall magnificent?' she asked him and without waiting for an answer continued, 'Despite the later additions I've always expected to see costumed figures walking out of it.' She spoke the last words almost to herself aware that her friend was not giving her his full attention.

Saxon was looking above him, into the sweeping branches of a Cedar of Lebanon. 'These are the fellows, I admire. Some say they were brought to England by the returning Crusaders, others say they were introduced as late as the sixteenth century. What do you think Beth?'

'Oh, by the Crusaders of course, far more romantic,' Elizabeth sighed and looked across to the flower beds in front of the hall. 'Don't you think these gardens are heavenly?' she asked him.

'They're alright I suppose. I say, do you think they'll be serving the grub soon?'

Elizabeth laughed. 'There will never be anyone like you Saxon, you're unique.'

In the salon the servants were uncovering the sumptuous buffet for which the Oakleys were well known. Robert, standing, close by the tables that spanned the top of the room, was in conversation with Victoria Burdette. He felt anything would be a welcome distraction from this girl he had been obliged to escort for the evening. How, he wondered, did she manage to speak almost normally with teeth like that? He stared at them again as if to punish himself, why they were almost horizontal.

Whilst appearing to listen, he allowed his attention to wander to the food, subconsciously checking the delicacies as each cloth was removed, he even found himself counting the home produce until he gave up, deciding that it practically all was, knowing as he did that their cook Mrs Wain was the envy of the county. Huge honey roast hams, pork pies, veal and ham pies with boiled eggs baked into them, cold sirloin of beef, pressed beasts tongues and other delicacies in aspic, plus a multitude of savoury tarts, green salads consisting of teens of ingredients, plump tomatoes and cheeses of every variety, all presented under the stare of a glazed boar's head.

'...and do you know Wobert, my thweet little spaniel girl, Dainty, is actuawally in our carriage at the moment. Wouldn't you just love to see her?'

Robert found himself smiling in agreement, anything, he felt would be preferable to standing about making small talk and listening to this inane prattle. 'After supper maybe.'

'Oh Wobert that would be lovely, I know she'll be so happy to meet you...' She continued to extol the virtues of her pet as Robert turned his eyes once more to the distraction the buffet offered.

There was, he was pleased to see, a good range of bottles, the cellars had given up admirably. Clusters of dusty bottles of red wine stood alongside great silver coolers filled with ice holding a varied selection of white wines. His pale eyes wandered to the tables beyond, more starched cloths displaying meringues, choux pastry delicacies of all kinds oozing with thick yellow cream, tiny pies decorated with pieces of glazed oranges, cherries and pineapple, Bakewell puddings, the whole colourful selection surmounted by huge bowls of exotic fruits from the hot houses around the walled garden. Robert could never remember being so interested in the presentation of a buffet. He turned back to Victoria once again and smiled wanly, then allowed his interest to stray out of the long windows and into the garden.

Guests were starting to make their way inside following Tomkins summons and between groups wandering into the salon Robert could see Saxon Brown sitting under the cedars talking to a girl in blue. He peered between guests who were making for the buffet tables. The girl was beautiful, how had he not noticed her before? From the distance he could see her glossy raven black hair, coiled at her neck with something glittering in it. Her face, was animated as she laughed at whatever that fool Brown was saying. Even from such a distance he could see her cheeks were flushed and she radiated health and vitality. As he watched, Saxon gave her his hand and helped her up offering his arm and as they started to walk across the lawn Robert saw that her figure was exquisite and the blue gown enhanced it to perfection.

'I say Victoria, sorry to interrupt but who's that girl with Saxon Brown? See, they're coming across the lawn now.'

Victoria stopped mid-sentence and squinted through the guests, 'Why don't you wecognise her Wobert? It's Elizabeth O'Malley Sullivan.'

Saxon held their plates aloft as he followed Elizabeth to a small table close by an entrance to the garden. Carefully he placed Elizabeth's supper in front of her. 'What shall I get you to drink Beth, there's champagne, any wine of your choice?'

'I'd like another glass of punch - it's really quite delicious.'

'Strong though,' Saxon warned, 'but then just what you need to brave dancing with me. Punch it shall be.' He crunched the two glasses into one hand and wandered off, self consciously pushing back his fair hair, causing it to stand on end. Elizabeth watching him, smiled fondly, he was, she thought, such a dear.

✹ ✹ ✹

Robert's eyes hadn't left Elizabeth, though to the most discerning observer he appeared to be devoting his entire attention to Miss Burdette. As Saxon left Elizabeth to fetch their drinks Robert made a move. He put his hand under the arm of his companion and steered her to the table where Elizabeth was seated. Her attention had been caught by a noisy party of some of her friends at the next table. Luke and Frederick Morley, sons of their doctor and Simon Lock the vicar's son, had involved Elizabeth in their conversation. She was so engrossed that Robert had to greet her for a second time.

Coughing pointedly he repeated himself, 'Elizabeth, sitting alone?'

Elizabeth smiled and stood to meet them, 'Oh no Robert, Saxon has just gone to fetch a glass of punch for me.' She indicated to the piled up plate opposite. 'He won't be many minutes.' Elizabeth laid her hand on the arm of the girl by Robert's side, 'Hello Victoria, how well you're looking and what a gorgeous gown.'

For the first time Robert really noticed what the girl he had been entertaining for almost an hour was wearing. He supposed it was rather fetching, obviously French, in shades of mauve. Hardly surprising he thought, as Victoria had just returned from Paris. The girls chatted politely as Robert watched. Their gowns, he was aware, clashed abominably, almost to a point where he considered he should not have brought them together. Neither was it just the gowns. He felt that Victoria, fair and petite, made a poor comparison next to Elizabeth, whose vital presence dominated the room, certainly for him. Why she made Victoria look practically invisible.

When, had this chrysalis turned into such a butterfly, he asked himself casting his mind back to the previous hunting season. Whilst he would admit that she always looked well turned out and could ride like no other, this dazzling creature was a different story altogether. He watched her closely as she spoke to Victoria, observing her small, even, white teeth between the most alluring lips he could recall seeing. She had the pert nose of many of Irish descent, a feature, the only feature, he would admit to admiring in the race and her eyes were the darkest blue he had ever seen. The floor shook, not, he told himself in irritation, by the effect Elizabeth O'Malley's eyes had upon him, but by the return of Saxon Brown, bearing two glasses.

'Hello Victoria, Robert,' Saxon grinned companionably as he put the drinks onto the table, spilling them a little. 'Can I fetch you anything whilst I'm at it?'

Robert shook his head, 'Actually Victoria and I will be eating shortly but she's not unnaturally anxious over her pet bitch left in the carriage. Knowing our stable staff I should think they are ruining the creature, but Victoria refuses to be consoled. I need to have a word with father on a small issue, so it may be a while before we manage supper if Victoria will be so accommodating as to wait for me.'

Saxon complied immediately with Robert's conniving.

'If Elizabeth is agreeable, we will accompany you to the stables whilst Robert's engaged with his family.'

Elizabeth nodded in agreement. 'Of course you must check your pet, how else will you enjoy the evening if you are concerned about her. Is it one of your King Charles spaniels?'

'Yes, Elizabeth, how clever of you to wemember.'

Robert glanced from one to the other and tightened his lips, 'You run along with Saxon my dear,' he told Victoria. 'There are one or two dates of meets that I would like to discuss with Elizabeth and then I really must see father.'

Saxon nodded to Elizabeth and offered his arm to Victoria. 'Shall we go then, see your little dog and put your mind at rest?'

Victoria hesitated for a moment, then smiled at Saxon, took his arm and allowed him to lead her from the room.

They had barely left before Elizabeth became thoroughly disenchanted by Robert's company. How ingratiating he had become, she decided and what of the dates he had mentioned? She had tried to steer the conversation back to what she considered to be the purpose of his company but as far as she could remember, there seemed to be no alterations to the dates already given for the following hunting season and she was feeling somewhat confused. Also she preferred that he wouldn't stand so near to her, his breath smelt strongly of whisky which she was finding quite repulsive, along with his glance which swept over her with a familiarity she resented. Elizabeth kept watch on the entrance to the salon as she nodded and made the odd comment, willing Saxon to return. She found herself wishing that the dancing would begin and smiled involuntarily at the thought, remembering the comments she had made to Saxon on their ride a few days ago.

'There my dear, I've got a smile from you and how charming it is.'

Elizabeth looked at him quizzically, her mind set on freeing herself as politely as possible. She took a step backwards and found herself against one of the fixed windows, Robert didn't miss the opportunity, he put his arm above her head and leaned his hand on the window frame, trapping her even closer to him than before.

'What do you say to a turn around the gardens to take some air before the dancing. Everyone seems to be inside now having supper, therefore we would have the grounds to ourselves.' He peered past her through the window. 'I see the gardeners have lit torches around the paths, it will be quite pleasant.'

Elizabeth ducked under his raised arm, 'I think not Robert, Saxon will be concerned as to where I am and I have promised to dance with him.'

'Tut tut my dear, he certainly cannot claim you for the entire evening, that would never do. You must spare time for your other old friends.' He smiled depreciatingly as Victoria and Saxon reappeared and crossed the room to join them.

'I am trying to convince Elizabeth that she must share her favours with all of her friends my dear chap, you have no right to keep her for yourself.' Robert smiled mischievously at Victoria as Saxon coloured up and began to stammer.

'I wouldn't dream of trying to monopolise Elizabeth, Robert, it's just that we're pals and I thought...' He shuffled his feet awkwardly and knocked the table sideways, Elizabeth had the forethought to move quickly but the freshly filled glasses of punch slewed sideways onto the front of Victoria's dress.

'Oh God I'm so sorry,' Saxon pulled at his handkerchief which Elizabeth noted was now tied around his hand and made to blot the gown but Victoria discouraged him.

'Please don't distress yourself Saxon, accidents will happen and I do feel bad about Dainty being so unkind to you so I beg of you not to give this a thought, I'll go up to the ladies cloakroom and see what the maid can do with it.'

How gracious she is, Elizabeth thought, warming towards the girl she already admired, 'I'll come with you Victoria,' and slipping her arm through Victoria's accompanied her from the room. Once they were out of sight, Robert turned on Saxon.

'You really are an offensive bugger, Brown. You ruin the gown of my companion and hog the best looking girl in the room.' Robert frowned at Saxon, 'I hope there's nothing between the two of you?' He didn't wait for an answer as he over ran himself, 'How that girl has changed, she's stunning, wasted on you if you don't mind my saying so. You're better sticking to racing and farming, surely even you can't get that wrong. And what happened with the damned dog? I expect you stood on it?'

'No I didn't, it just took a dislike to me and bit my hand.'

'The creature was lucky it wasn't me, I would have throttled the bloody thing. I remember throttling a puppy as a child, came over loathing it.'

Saxon glared at him in disgust, but Robert was only interested in his own flow of words.

'Victoria seems to be obsessed with those blasted dogs, it's pathetic. There's one thing about Elizabeth O'Malley Sullivan, she's got her priorities right, horses count for everything with her.' He stared at the young man, engaging Saxon's bright blue eyes with his own pale ones and lowering his voice, said, 'I could change that if I so choose and choose I might.'

⚭ ⚭ ⚭

Elizabeth was silent in the carriage on the return journey. Her parents, seated opposite were discussing the evening and having unsuccessfully tried to involve her in their conversation left her in peace to her thoughts, which had they known, were not happy ones. Elizabeth reflected upon the evening, which had been a disappointment to her. It had been spoilt from the point where Robert Oakley had joined them and chosen to monopolise her. She frowned, was she imagining that? No, for he had been quite persistent, even to the point of intruding on them during the dancing and ushering Saxon in Victoria's direction. She shuddered, recalling Robert's sour breath on her cheek and clammy hands even through the cotton gloves he wore. Some protection for her gown, she thought. She put her hand to her forehead, feeling the coolness of her fingers easing the tension that had built up behind her eyes which were beginning to sting with tears as she recalled Saxon's bewilderment and Victoria's hurt.

V

Elizabeth could not sleep. It seemed hours since they had returned from the ball. Through the slender posts of her bed she could see the blue gown laid across a chair, shimmering in the moonlight which flooded through the window and cast the square glazing bars into long shadows. Events of the evening revolved around her head causing her senses to reel with disgust as she recalled again, the sight and worse, the odour of Robert Oakley. What could he want of her? She already knew that Victoria Burdette had been earmarked for him and a sweeter girl she felt would be difficult to imagine, added to this, Elizabeth had noticed during the evening that Victoria was not averse to Robert, making the embarrassment she had felt by his attentions to her, even worse. Contrarily, in the past, he had shown no interest in her whatsoever except to torment her, along with his sisters. Elizabeth shuddered, remembering the panic she had felt, when he had trapped her against the window earlier that evening.

She tossed and turned trying to shut out the memories of Robert's behaviour and her endeavours to understand it. Eventually she got out of bed and looked down on the top yard. She loved her room at the side of the house, which afforded this outlook and from the open window listened to the familiar sounds, the scrape of an iron shoe on the blue bricks of the stable floor, the sound of a horse blowing down its nostrils, the rattle of a chain from the stalls. The moon's pale rays bathed the yard in soft light. She sank down onto the window seat and rested her head against the shutters folded against the wall, raising her knees and wrapping her arms around them. The peace and security of her home surroundings began to work their charm and the familiarity of the yard below was balm to her. How delicate was the moon wash on the gravel, no earthly colour could be compared with it. Glancing to her right the beech and oak trees stood reassuringly sentinel some distance behind the stack yard.

Her eyes strayed back towards the roofs of the buildings in the top yard, when a light attracted her attention for a second and then was gone. Could it have been the reflection of the moon on a skylight? She strained her eyes for a while but it was no longer visible, someone she thought must have walked by a skylight in the loft with a lantern. Was there trouble with one of the horses? Or could there be a more sinister reason for the light? Swiftly she dressed in breeches and a shirt, then quietly made her way to the postern door collecting her boots on the way. She let herself out of the house silently, whispering to Major and Dolcis, the yard dogs who had come out of their kennels to investigate, then walked on the edge of the gravel, her feet making no sound.

Noiselessly she let herself into the stables through the yard door the top half of which was kept open. When closing the bottom half, she scraped the bolt slightly, attracting Minette's welcoming whinny. Too late for her presence to be unknown, she stood quietly in the shadows of the passageway in front of the loose boxes and stalls, her heartbeats seemingly so loud in her ears that they would give her away. A shaft of moonlight illuminated a large square on the passage floor in front of the half door and smaller patches from the barred windows ranged each side of it. The loft stairs were in darkness, but Elizabeth's eyes were becoming accustomed to this and she kept her eyes upon them. After some seconds she heard a movement, from the top step a boot appeared followed by another, then a pair of cord breeches and green shirt, then the face she knew so well.

'James,' she whispered, 'you scared me, I saw the light from my room. Is anything wrong?'

He came down the last of the wooden steps and stood facing her. 'I don't know Beth, you tell me, I haven't settled all night, not since you left for the hall.'

How like the old days, she thought, for him to know instinctively that she was disturbed, yet for once, in view of his dislike of Robert, caution advised her to disclose nothing of the evening's events.

'Someone's upset you?'

'No.'

'Someone at the ball?'

'No.'

He moved nearer and looked into her face through the semi darkness, Elizabeth knew he was trying to glean from her expression the cause of his concern for her. She felt his closeness starting to have the same effect as it had in the meadow just a few weeks before, her legs beginning to feel as though they no longer belonged to her and she found herself swaying towards him. She flinched as his hands gripped her upper arms, his strength flooding into her. One of the horses pawed at the bedding, another paused from chewing hay for a moment and a yard dog gave a solitary bark. The familiar sounds seemed distant and unreal.

'Beth,' his voice was low and urgent, 'are you alright?'

His breath fanned her cheek and she leaned further towards him, aching with longing to be close to him.

'Beth, do you know what you're doing?'

'Hold me James, hold me tight.'

He relinquished his grip on her arms and drew her to him. Elizabeth clung to him and lay her head in the side of his neck breathing in his wholesomeness, he smelt of soap and the hay in which he had been lying. She turned her face to him and met his eyes. For some time they gazed at each other, then James seemed to wake as if from sleep. He put his hands on her shoulders and backed away from her, 'I've left a lamp in the loft, I must fetch it down before we leave.'

He turned and made his way up the steps. Elizabeth stared after him in bewilderment, her arms dropped by her sides and she gasped, fighting back tears. Then, impulsively she ran up the steps and followed him into the loft. He had snuffed out the lamp and stood with it in his hand. A wisp of smoke unfurled towards a skylight and was lost in the small moonlit pane. They faced each other in its pale light.

'You pushed me away...' she covered her face with her hands and sank down on the hay, 'am I so repulsive to you?' She could feel hot tears running between her fingers as humiliation overcame her insecurity.

James hung the lamp on the beam and sat close beside her, 'Repulsive? You mean more to me than anything.' He took her hands from her face and lifted her chin forcing her to look at him. Elizabeth raised her eyes to his, tears spilling down her cheeks. James' voice was husky and intense, 'I can't imagine life without you, I never could. But now...'

His grey eyes held hers and she felt a knot in her abdomen.

'Now...' he rubbed his hand roughly across his forehead, 'you're so beautiful Beth. You always have been to me, but things have changed between us, we're both different. You know it too, the afternoon in the hayfield was when we both discovered each other as we are now, isn't that true?'

She nodded miserably, 'Am I wrong to want you to hold me in your arms?'

'No, not wrong, but maybe not wise?'

'What's wisdom got to do with it?'

'Beth can't you see I'm trying to do what's right and it's not easy for me.'

'I know what's right for us James, as you do, I understand you so well that your thoughts are my thoughts.' She lifted her hand to his face and traced her finger gently along his mouth.

Slowly, so slowly that a shiver of anticipation rippled through her, he bent his head and brushed his lips against hers. From deep inside her a longing for him caused her to part her lips and offer her mouth to him tenderly then almost fiercely as they fell back into the hay and she felt the wonderful weight of him crushing her so that she could scarcely breath and felt that she was becoming part of him.

✤ ✤ ✤

In the weeks that followed, Elizabeth and James lived in an ecstatic, unforgettable world of their own. They ignored the rumblings of a troubled world, living only for the present, which was theirs for the taking. The loft became their haven and they spent many hours in each other's arms. Their work did not suffer for they put as much into their days as ever and in their hands the young horses promised to be amongst the finest the O'Malley Stud had produced.

Already John had been approached by a number of reputable trainers interested to buy young hunter-chasers for their owners. Their work did not go unnoticed by John and Tom, neither did their closeness. John was beginning to think that Elizabeth would benefit from a stay with Mary's elder widowed sister, Martha, in Lincoln. The matter would have been settled, but Doctor Morley had reluctantly informed John that Mary's health was declining and he had no wish to share his concerns with her at such a time, particularly as Mary was blissfully unaware of Elizabeth's interest outside horses. It was not long however, before Tom, shared his fears with Annie.

Reclining in his favourite position on the black oak settle which flanked the kitchen range, Tom stared up at the rows of polished horse brasses on the beams. His family had been with horses for many years and the collection of brasses had belonged to his father who had shown fine Shires, Mighty Hawker, Canute, Iron Mask and the likes. Amongst the brasses, bunches of dried herbs loaned their fragrance to Tom's nostalgic thoughts. He transferred his gaze to his wife seated opposite to him, she was busying herself with a pile of mending, her eyes screwed up behind the wire spectacles she had recently acquired, sorting lengths of wool in the flickering light of the oil lamp. On her knee was one of James' jerseys. James, the son they had never had. Tom thought back to the day they'd brought him home when Annie's younger sister and her husband had taken so desperately ill. It had been no less than a miracle that the child hadn't followed his parents to the grave. Tom's face softened as he thought of Margaret and Joseph Gretton, lost to their son who had become everything to him and Annie. He frowned as the anxiety which was troubling him flooded back into his mind.

He broached the subject. 'Where's James, Annie?'

'With the horses I should think, where else would he be?' she squinted her eyes as she threaded a bodkin. 'I've never known a boy more devoted to horses than James, that's thanks to you Tom, you've been a better father to him than many are to their own.' She smiled fondly across at him.

'I think with Elizabeth would be more like it.' He waited for her reaction.

'Well, what's new about that? Haven't they always worked together? I've always thought it's really nice how John and Mary have accepted their friendship, no sooner had the two of them learned to walk than they were inseparable, never far away from each other.'

Tom studied the herringbone brick floor, 'What if it's become more than friendship Annie?'

He sensed rather than saw her lay down her darning, 'Tom, what are you saying?' Her smile faltered as she peered at him.

'Anybody who sees them together these days Annie would wonder. John does I'm sure of that, but he's got plenty on with Mary being so poorly an' all.'

Annie shook her head sadly, 'Poor lady, I truly think she's the gentlest and kindest person I've ever known.' She took off her glasses and wiped the corners of her eyes.

'Aye, she is that, but did you hear what I was telling you about the two of 'em?'

'We've agreed haven't we that they've always been close?'

'Annie, you know full well what I'm trying to get over to you, you're stalling. It's got to be faced, we've got a situation here and I for one don't like it.'

'You can't mean what you're saying. I know the family are unusual how they've brought Elizabeth up, I mean, she's always had so much freedom to come and go as she pleases, mix with all the stable hands and come here like a second home,' she laughed. 'No Tom, I think you're wrong, they've always been the best of friends especially as they're both on their own, so what if they do stick together. They'll go their own separate ways in the course of time, you mark my words. Now don't you worry yourself about it any more, you're being fanciful that's all.'

But Tom wasn't so sure, he sighed as he watched Annie resume mending James' jersey, then picking up *The Nottingham Evening Post,* read of the ongoing unrest across Europe.

❧ ❧ ❧

Whilst Tom was expressing his concerns to Annie, John was dining at the hall along with most of his male counterparts in and around Oakley.

Ralph's guests seated at a large mahogany table were, John, Charles Burdette, Doctor Andrew Morley and his two sons Luke and Frederick, the Reverend Lock and his son Simon, Richard Brown and sons Edward and Saxon, and Robert Oakley. The party, who had already imbibed freely in the library at the insistence of Ralph were enjoying Mrs Wain's excellent selection of *hors d'oeuvre* followed by her speciality, *consommé vert,* and were absorbed in frank discussion on the serious situation escalating across Europe. Tomkins super-vised the serving of the *fillets de soles à la meuniere,* refilling glass-es himself with a well chilled *muscadet,* as conversation became more animated. John leaned back in his chair absently observing Ralph's butler who never failed to anticipate the needs of a guest and who when the previous course had been cleared, raised his gloved hand in the direction of a footman who disappeared momentarily and returned wheeling a great rolled top silver meat dish which Tomkins opened with a flourish to reveal a splendid joint of sirloin.

'Ah, the beef,' Ralph beamed genially around his friends.

John nudged him, 'Go on Ralph tell us.'

There was an expectant hush around the table.

'The finest beef in the world, got to be, for wasn't the loin knight-ed by James the First. Marbled beef from the White Cattle, the old-est breed in Britain, a herd of which have roamed across the parkland of Oakley for centuries.'

The assembly cheered, they heard Ralph extolling the virtues of his beloved cattle whenever beef was served at his dinners, yet never tired of listening, knowing that all he said was true and they tucked their napkins into their necks in anticipation.

'Can't think why you don't reinstate a herd Charles,' Ralph told Charles Burdette.

'I expect you'll wear me down eventually,' Charles answered. He explained to the group, 'Forefathers ran a big herd of White Cattle at Lowerton, as you may know. Yew killed them in the seventeen hundreds, blasted yew saw them all off, by all accounts it must have been terrible.'

'Lethal stuff, best confined to churchyards and enclosed gardens,' Reverend Lock said, shaking his head.

'Must say you're doing us damned proud Ralph,' Andrew Morley remarked as he was served a generous portion of beef. From around the table there were similar comments of appreciation.

Ralph nodded, unashamedly pleased by the compliment. 'The cloud under which we are living is getting darker, what better than to be with one's friends at such a time.' His face was reddened by the heat of the room exacerbated by the flickering heat of a myriad of candles illuminating the table for although he had seen to it that the hall was now lit by electricity he still preferred candlelight when entertaining. 'More intimate eh, keeps those around the table isolated from the rest of the room, like an island, don't you know,' he would frequently tell his wife when she was planning their dinners. He now pointed his finger around the table indicating to one of the footman serving vegetables. 'Plenty now, see that you give 'em plenty, can't beat vegetables to keep a man's innards healthy.'

Robert rolled up his eyes at Saxon seated opposite.

'Fine vegetables they look Ralph,' the Reverend Lock commented, 'home grown I'll be bound.'

Ralph beamed, 'They certainly are George, all from our own gardens.'

Tomkins was pouring claret from one of a group of cut glass decanters which stood together against the green curtain on the back of a large sideboard.

'Decanted the claret myself, took me best part of the afternoon, worth it though.' Ralph laughed dryly, 'Put down by my father in the fifties, I think he'd come back and haunt me if I didn't decant it exactly as he taught me, candle behind the flow. Got it off to a fine art, haven't we Tomkins, best part of the damned afternoon I tell you, but worth it, let's see.' He held his glass to the flame in front of him, 'See, clear as a ruby, beautiful.' He looked hard at the younger men seated around the table, 'Make it your business to decant claret properly, skill that will last you a lifetime.'

Conversation was stilled temporarily whilst the excellent beef received their full attention, then gradually resumed, voices rising and falling. Inevitably, the impending threat of war was uppermost in their minds.

'Why,' Edward Brown reasoned, 'though absolutely appalling, should the assassinations of the Grand Archduke Frans Ferdinand and his wife, throw the whole of Europe into turmoil?'

Ralph answered him, 'Bosnian Slavs, Austrian subjects, have been spoiling for trouble for years Edward and they see the assassination of an Austrian by a Serb Nationalist as a challenge to Austrian rule over Serbia.'

There was general agreement as the vicar spoke up, 'God forbid we are thrown into war again, but I agree with Ralph, Austria seem determined aggressors, and now they have the full support of Germany...' He shook his head.

'The Kaiser is unpredictable at the best of times and these certainly are not amongst them,' Andrew Morley intervened glancing around the table.

'Germany is glad of the opportunity to get involved if you ask me,' Robert adding, 'blindly following that little prig Wilhelm.'

Saxon spoke up, 'What about Russia, I would have thought involvement was the last thing the Russian people would want?'

'Russia will support Serbia,' Charles Burdette said. 'Their involvement is inevitable.'

'Russia's already got troubles of her own brewing there,' Ralph glanced from one to the other.

'When you think of what they endured a hundred years ago, their victory over the French was little short of a miracle.' Simon Lock interjected. 'The terrible sacrifices of the ordinary people. All sides are losers in war, the prospect doesn't bear thinking about.'

There were assents around the table. Frederick, Doctor Morley's younger son said thoughtfully, 'I can understand the reasons for anger and urge to defend if our families and way of life are threatened, but does any of this present a threat to us?'

His father, turned to him, 'I fear that the threat is already hanging over us Frederick, along with the rest of Europe, who like us, are reluctant to take up arms against the Austrian Germany cause, but we must be prepared to go to the defence of our allies and I don't think it will be long coming.'

There were nods of agreement as Andrew Morley had voiced what they all knew to be true. Richard Brown steered the conversation around to his own eminent field, the Boer War and of Field Marshall Lord Roberts with whom he had served, speaking passionately of his admiration for the man.

John remained silent, he still felt a twinge of guilt concerning that war and whenever he was reminded of it, anger arose inside him. Mary and he were married in 1896 and in 1899 at the outbreak, Elizabeth was little more than a baby and Mary's health was causing anxiety. He had then as now been up to the neck in the affairs of the stud and he didn't go. Hell, he had other things to do. He was damned if he was going to sacrifice his family and his business, feeling as he had at the beginning of the war that the cause was aggravated by crowds of grasping gold diggers after the Transvaal find. John toyed with his cheese, absently accepting the port as it circulated around the table. His thoughts were interrupted by Ralph.

'My friends, I fear we have bad times coming, the way events are heading could well turn Europe upside down. Our way of life as we know it could be changed forever. We must come through this as best we can, tighten the bonds of family and friends and call on the fortitude of the nation. Should the appalling predictions come to pass, those of us around this table who are too old to take up the sword will reluctantly pass it on to our sons. May God help them.'

The port had given way to brandy. Ralph waited until the glasses of his guests had been charged, then he rose, 'Gentlemen please join me in a toast,' he raised his glass as they all stood. 'The King.'

'The King,' the company repeated.

A little later, the diners bearing their glasses, straggled through into the library, Ralph's favourite retreat, all but the Reverend Lock who gave his apologies and made to leave, hustling his son before him, 'Early start you know Sunday, nature of the job.' The other guests laughed on cue having heard the witticism many times. After Ralph had sent a footman to the stables to have the vicar's carriage brought round and seen his guests off, the party settled at card tables.

'Mixed ages, I insist,' Ralph called, selecting a cigar proffered by Tomkins.

The party made up three tables consisting of two threes and a four. John found himself on a table of three along with Doctor Morley and Robert Oakley. The players at the tables gradually became immersed as they peered through what was becoming a haze of tobacco smoke. Brandy glasses were topped and re-topped and Robert who'd had surprising little to contribute to the conversation at dinner, now came into his own. Holding a brandy glass aloft he leaned back in his chair and surveyed John almost impertinently.

'You undoubtedly must feel quite at home sir, at a card game.'

John chose to ignore the inflexion in Robert's voice. 'Indeed Robert, there is little I enjoy more than a good game.' He commenced dealing, yet even before he had done so Robert spoke again, like a terrier, John thought, with a bone it would not release.

'No doubt your ancestor felt the same way when he left here with some of our land.'

John sighed, he had, over the years been chaffed by Ralph over the folly of their respective grandfathers, but he hardly expected it from his son whose manner he felt quite lacked the good natured ribbing he had taken without offence from Ralph.

He refused, however to be drawn and keeping his eyes on his hand of cards answered levelly, 'His land Robert, he won it fair and square.'

Robert indicated the pile of sovereigns and half sovereigns on the table. 'A few sovereigns are what you win fair and square in a game, not the next best farm on the estate.'

John continued to study his hand. 'It was a different age, with different values. Why, fortunes could be won and lost in those days over a game of cards. It was common practice. Both of our forebears were gambling men by all accounts, it's well known in our family that my grandfather put up his horses and his place in Derbyshire, all he had in fact. I fear there was little to pick between them, they both knew what they were doing.'

'Perhaps one day sir, you'll give me the opportunity to win it back?'

'I think not Robert, we O'Malley's have learned to be less reckless over the years.' John caught Andrew Morley's eye and smiled, seeing the doctor relax, but not before he had caught an expression he could only have described as malice on the face of Robert Oakley.

VI

AUGUST 1914

Elizabeth and James were oblivious to the concern they were causing to their families. Throughout June and July they had ridden the young horses out in pairs each day. It didn't go unnoticed that their rides were becoming longer and longer as the summer progressed.

At the beginning of August they decided to take a whole day to enjoy their favourite ride. James was the first down to the stables and was already grooming Rua when Elizabeth slipped quietly into the passageway. She hesitated upon hearing James' voice and though she couldn't decipher what he was saying, was aware he was speaking to the stallion. His voice was soft and low and as she heard no movement from the horse, knew that the animal was listening to James' soothing tone as he worked.

In that moment Elizabeth felt a bizarre tightness in her chest, almost as though invisible threads had reached out to her, irreversibly tying the three of them together with the strangest and most inexplicable force.

'Beth, is that you?' She heard James speak her name but stood for a moment, powerless to move, disturbed by the fleeting experience which had gripped her only seconds before.

'Beth, are you alright?'

Elizabeth blinked hard, finding that James was holding her forearms, shaking her slightly and looking at her intently.

She stared at him, then, reality returning, smiled into his eyes, 'How could I be any other darling James, with the prospect of spending a whole day close to you.'

'You seemed to be miles away.'

'I was with you on another plane.'

He pulled a face. 'Welcome back to this one,' he kissed her light-ly on the mouth. 'I've groomed the gelding and practically finished Rua,' he grinned conspiringly inclining his head to the window sill of the passageway. 'See I got some sandwiches and a flask of water.'

'Same here, I talked cook into making some of those lovely thin bacon sandwiches we eat on the way back from hunting and what's more,' she told him in a low voice, 'I've borrowed Papa's flask and filled it with port wine, it really will be like the delicious combination we have on hunt days.'

James laughed, 'You're pushing the boat out Beth.'

'Why not?' she said, placing her booty by the side of his. 'Come on let's tack up and get off before the lads start to arrive.'

In the tack room she stayed his hand as he reached for her side saddle. 'No, James, I'm riding astride, be damned to convention. Why, one of the Misses Deerham Majors' rode in the Earl of Harrington's point to point astride last Easter, so I'm sure I can.'

'In that case even more reason why we should be away from the village before any of Oakley tittle tattlers are abroad and also Pa's questions about where we're going and how long we'll be.'

'I told Papa we were taking Rua and another of the youngsters for a good long ride they could really enjoy after all their hard work.'

'Finest thing out for them,' James agreed as he saddled up the stal-lion.

'Papa didn't ask which ride we are going, but truly no one takes much notice where I am or what I'm doing at the moment with Mama ill. When I'm not with her that is, but when I am, I read to her, or we just talk. She loves to reminisce about the days when I was small and we had picnics together and she taught me the names of wild flowers. Mama is the dearest of all human beings.'

'She is that,' James said with feeling as they led the horses out onto the gravel and mounted.

They turned west from the yard, the sun behind them, the air balmy and still. A wide grass verge silenced the iron shod hooves until they turned north into the bridle road which crossed the fields to Springleigh, Kelingleigh and into Nuthall, well known for its Palladian Temple by the lake. Riding past the ancient church of St. Patrick they turned left, on through Watnall past the Royal Oak and blacksmith's shop amongst a cluster of cottages. Side by side they rode through Greasley, to their left the ancient remains of Greasley Castle and square tower of the church, to their right the Victorian Rectory, standing high above its apron of paddock.

The headstocks were already turning at Moorgreen colliery and the rhythmic beat of the steam winder could be heard across the village where the gardens of strung out cottages were still bright with flowers in spite of the lack of rain all summer. They turned off to the right passing the red lodge and into a bridle path through a wood, countryside which had quietly witnessed the first and lasting love of Lord Byron.

Elizabeth closed her eyes and breathed in the aroma of the wood, identifying the mixture of earth and crushed leaf mould disturbed by the horses' hooves and the scent of dead bracken under the fading summer growth.

'This is heaven,' she told James reaching for his hand. 'I've such happy memories of this ride over the years. Do you remember when the elders would bring us here as children, they considered it would be an endurance test for us. How wrong they were, we loved every minute of it didn't we? I can see us now riding through here eating those floury baps cook made and biting into tomatoes from the glass house. We had floury moustaches and squirted tomato seeds over our clothes and down the horses' manes.' She laughed, 'What messy little devils we were. Happy though.'

'We've shared a lot, Beth, we took it for granted when we were younger, I know I did. How many employers would involve the family of an employee as your father does?'

'Tom's more than that to the stud, for goodness sake. Papa depends on him.'

James shrugged, 'You know what I mean.'

'Come on let's give the horses a run for their money, the going's perfect here, not dried out as most of the ground is.'

They urged the horses first into a canter and still well in hand pressed them to gallop on, holding them neck and neck, stride for stride. The trees flashed by and a minute dot of light appeared in the distance. They raced towards it, muscles of horses and riders stretched with effort. The light became a shaft and the end of the tunnel of trees drew nearer.

They reined the horses as they burst into the sunlight and walked them up the ascent from the valley, riding close their legs touching and from time to time James reached out to her, to stroke her cheek, push back her hair or ride with his hand on her shoulder. Elizabeth felt she could explode with happiness. Each time James looked at her, touched her, she was filled with a longing for him, an aching which she found both disturbing and pleasing.

James resumed their earlier conversation. 'We've known each other all our lives, do you realise that, Beth?'

'We have, yet you seem to be quite different from those days, suddenly our lives have changed, they have changed haven't they, James?'

He reached for her hand, 'More than I thought possible. Imagine what we could have missed.'

'I couldn't bear to,' she told him. 'I feel part of you. I only want to be with you day and night.'

'Hush, you sound shameless and you're not, let's keep what we have close to us and value it while we have it.'

'James,' Elizabeth reined her horse, 'James, how could you say that or even think it. We're destined to be together always now.'

He put his hand under her chin, 'I hope so, Beth, I really and truly hope so.' She looked hard into his face, reassured by the sincerity in his eyes.

He dug deep into the pocket of his breeches, 'I want you to have this, it means a lot to me. It's all I have of my father's. I understand that it's been in the family for a long time. An ancestor of ours made the pilgrimage to Santiago de Compostella, to the tomb of St. James. Annie told me that it was given to me at my baptism, passed on to me for my name.'

He held up a medallion on a silver chain and reached out of the saddle and placed it over her head.

She felt the weight settle on her shirt before she lifted it up to examine it. 'Why James, it's beautiful, the shape of a cockleshell, emblem of the Compostella pilgrimage.' She felt her eyes beginning to sting. 'I've never known anyone who's made that journey,' she held the medallion in her hand. 'How can I take it from you?'

'Because I love you and while ever you wear it I shall believe that you love me.'

'I'll always love you, James. I'll love you until I die.' The threatened tears spilled from her eyes as she studied his face.

He stroked her wet cheek. 'It will be a bond between us, wear it for me.'

She nodded and slipped the medallion under her shirt next to her skin feeling the warmth of him still on it and she dashed the tears from her eyes as she looked back at him 'I vow to St. James before God that I'll never take it off.'

They had reached the top of the hill, a ruined cottage stood by a cart track and an old but stout gate still guarded the overgrown path. They dismounted, slackened the girths and sat on the gate, reins loosely held whilst the horses pulled at long strands of dry grass. To their left an abandoned farm cart lay, crooked for want of a wheel, its shafts lost in tufts of faded grass and to the right by James, a long forgotten damask rose overhung a crumbling wall.

Elizabeth shaded her eyes against the sun and gazed down the valley. The hot, dry summer had taken its toll and the fields which rolled out below them were brown and shrivelled, though the hedges still retained their colour and stretched out in green precision around the fields they enclosed. James leaned over and broke off a rose twisting the stalk around in his fingers as his eyes swept across the valley.

Elizabeth watched him toying with the rose, his hands fascinating her as they always did, tanned with short cut nails, strong, yet gentle with the flower. He turned from the view and handed the rose to her. She held it to her nose and breathed in its heady fragrance, then held it to his face for him to do the same. He laughed and took it from her, carefully weaving it into the buttonhole of her shirt. She felt almost faint by his nearness and raising her head to meet his, leaned towards him as he caught her with his arm about her and kissed her gently on the mouth.

They almost overbalanced but James jumped down pulling her with him. The horses started for a moment but resumed grazing as James pressed her to the gate, bent his head and kissed her again, their bodies fusing in the embrace. Elizabeth felt dizzy as his kisses gained urgency. The restlessness of the horses brought them to reality and James looking into her eyes breathed deeply and grinned at her, shaking his head at the animals. He tightened the girths, cupped his hands and threw her up onto the gelding, even placing her feet in the stirrups. Elizabeth, as if helpless, let him, knowing that if anyone but he had tried this, she would have remonstrated strongly. They rode across the plateau towards Annesley forest. Elizabeth sighed contentedly as she returned James' gaze, seeing that his eyes held the same intensity of feeling as her own.

In the forest the foresters had left a huge pile of trunks across one of the rides off to the left. James jerked his head in the direction of it. Elizabeth nodded. Simultaneously they turned the horses and rode them hard towards the obstacle. They took off together and flew over the jump, then cantered on up the ride to find more of the stacked trunks, setting the horses at them as they thundered through the wide grassy ride. Then, of the same mind they turned and took the jumps back, returning to the pathway, breathless and exhilarated sharing the satisfaction of well schooled horses with the heart to do what was asked of them without hesitation.

'They were perfect,' Elizabeth shouted to James, slowing the gelding into a walk.

'Perfect schooling,' James agreed, his face breaking into a grin. 'The people responsible must be brilliant.'

Elizabeth stood in her stirrups. 'Brilliant, gifted and in love with each other, horses and life,' she shouted the words and listened for the echo.

'And with this day too, long may they remember it,' James' echo chased Elizabeth's around the still woodland and the laughter which followed it. Once back on the road through the forest, James turned round fiddling with the canvas lunch bag he had tied to 'D' rings on the saddle. He manipulated it onto his knee and pulled out thick cut sandwiches bursting with home cured ham, passing one to Elizabeth.

'Gorgeous, Annie's best,' Elizabeth closed her eyes as she tore at the bread, mustard oozing over the ham.

He nodded as he chewed. 'No one can cure ham like Ma. I love to eat a picnic riding, needs must, you either eat as you ride or dismount and be persecuted to death.'

Elizabeth laughed. 'Too true, anyway I don't like tit bitting horses, it can make them nappy and disagreeable. Except Rua, he's too much of a gentleman to seek out treats, he prefers them left quietly in the manger.' She fanned her sandwich at a cloud of flies which were following them. 'I didn't realise I was so hungry,' Elizabeth spoke with her mouth full, 'I didn't have any breakfast, did you?'

'No, I'm starving. Let's be having those thin bacon ones now and some port, the water can wait.'

❧ ❧ ❧

It was very late when Elizabeth and James returned to the stud. Elizabeth felt her stomach churn as they turned in the gates, envisaging her father's reaction to the hours they had been absent. It was not her father who came out of the stables to help untack the horses, it was Tom. Elizabeth saw at once that his face was grave.

They learned that the country had been at war since eleven o'clock the previous evening. It was Wednesday, 5th August, 1914.

PART TWO

REALITY

*The crimes of war
are not restricted
to the battlefield.*

Anonymous, 1914

VII

Robert rode into the bottom yard of the O'Malley stables. Had he set out to make the maximum impact he could hardly have timed it better. James was leading Rua out to go with the second lot for exercise. The yard was filling with geldings who exercised with the entires. Lads were bustling about whilst John and Tom were leaning over the wall by the yard pump discussing some young stock they needed to get to Kelingleigh station on the first leg of their journey to Ireland. Elizabeth, in shabby breeches and open neck blue shirt was by Rua's head talking to James.

The bustle turned to tableau as glances turned in Robert's direction. He had recently taken up a commission and was immaculately turned out in a newly tailored uniform. From his highly polished brown boots and Sam Brown belt, to his cap, he looked every inch the part. He beckoned with his cane to one of the lads, 'My horse.'

He dismounted and made his way to Elizabeth. 'My dear, I couldn't leave for Sandhurst without saying goodbye to you, perhaps you can spare a little of your time for an old friend?'

Elizabeth's flushed, 'Why... yes of course Robert. Will you come into the house, we've had breakfast between first and second exercise but I'm sure cook can make us tea.'

'How delightful,' he stood back to allow her to lead him up to the house noticing as he did so that she exchanged a glance with the lad who held the red stallion. Robert narrowed his eyes and scrutinised James as he passed him, he was sure the lad was the foundling who had been reared on the place, something to do with the stud groom he recalled, probably some by-blow he'd got lumbered with. He'd never liked the creature around Elizabeth, or their easy familiarity, but the look he had just caught passing between them caused his face to blanch with fury. Why, it was almost as though she needed the wretch's approval to leave the yard.

By the time they had reached the house he had recovered himself, dismissing his suspicions. Perish the thought, he should have known better, for despite their eccentricity, the O'Malley family did at least have some sense of propriety.

Elizabeth offered Robert a seat in the drawing room and dashed to the kitchen where their cook was seated at the pine scrubbed table earnestly writing in her recipe book, glasses perched on the end of her nose. She looked up as Elizabeth burst through the door. 'Lord a mercy Miss Elizabeth whatever's the matter?'

'Oh nothing's wrong Mrs. Bailey. Robert Oakley has called and I wondered if we could have some tea?'

Mrs. Bailey got to her feet. 'Of course and some of my poppy seed cake, I've just made a fresh one, I know how much you like it.'

'You're a dear,' Elizabeth's words were trapped in the door as she rushed out of the kitchen and into the passageway. Once outside the baize door she stopped for a moment, knowing that she should change. What if he thought she was making an effort for him? Never, she thought with a shudder, yet her mother's gentle disapproval should she sit in the drawing room in stable clothes rankled her conscience and swiftly she dived back through the passageway into the mud room and changed into the simple dark blue skirt and blouse that she had worn for breakfast. After washing her hands and smoothing her skirt she joined Robert, finding that Mrs. Bailey had already had Jenna, the parlour maid, set a tray of tea before him.

'My dear, you look charming. I must say I was somewhat disconcerted by your former appearance.' He took the cup Elizabeth offered to him and helped himself to a large spoonful of sugar. 'We really must see what can be done to persuade you to do a little less work. Ride, Elizabeth, by all means ride, no one looks finer on a horse than you do and let those your father pays get on with the rest.' He accepted a piece of seed cake absently as he warmed to his subject,

'Particularly now you are getting older, you must take care to avoid any form of familiarity with those in the yards or you could find it very difficult to discourage, mark my words.' A superior smile played about his lips. 'There is an old saying, familiarity breeds contempt, don't allow anyone to be either familiar or contemptuous towards you my dear, far better to be aloof than find you have to come down with a heavy hand, don't you think?'

'Heavy hand, whatever do you mean?'

Robert leaned back in the chair, his pale eyes on her face. 'There are ways my dear, but nothing for you to worry your pretty head about.'

Elizabeth frowned. 'The way in which Papa runs our business, Robert, has always been successful, he considers the people who work here to be no less than himself. It's his way and it works well.' She took his cup to refill it, adding, 'Our horses are renowned throughout this country, Ireland and in more recent years, the continent. We must be doing something right.'

He smiled disarmingly, 'I trust by we you do not use the royal form but mean your father and yourself?'

'And those who work with us.'

'For you, Elizabeth.'

'With us Robert.'

Robert felt his frustration mounting, this was really not the atmosphere he had intended, far from it, he had hoped to make an impression on her, this being his first outing in uniform. Elizabeth was aware of the tension between them and was at a loss to know what could have caused his displeasure. Surely not her relationship with everyone on the place? Why the teamwork at the O'Malley stud was well known and respected throughout horse breeding circles. It must be apprehension for what lay ahead, she decided, the daunting prospect of facing the unknown and tried to imagine how she herself would feel in the same circumstances.

As if reading of her thoughts, Robert reached to a side table with magazines scattered upon it and picked out the *Nottingham Evening*

Post from the previous day.

Wounded coming home in hundreds, he read aloud, *Hearty recep-tions. Country houses for convalescent. Germans advance on Compiegne forty miles from Paris.* He turned the page apparent-ly looking for something else and with a covert glance at her, read out: *Horses for cavalry and light draft horses are still urgently needed for the British forces. Major A. W. Waite who is purchas-ing animals for the War Office in this district says there has been a fair amount of business doing and some animals of excellent quality have been offered for purchase. Many hunting gentlemen in the vicinity have, with real public spirit offered the whole of their horses, but the supply falls short of the demand and it is ani-mals of the hunter type which are needed most.*

He closed the paper and returned it to the magazine pile. 'These types of advertisements are in the *Post* every day now.'

Elizabeth shook her head sadly. 'It's unbelievable how many horses the army are buying. There are train loads of them at all of the local stations. Papa is having a difficult time trying to get some of the horses we have sold to their destinations.'

Robert was not to be easily deflected. 'Mark my words, this is just the beginning Elizabeth, you've seen nothing yet, when the source of buying horses dries up the army will commandeer.'

'Commandeer,' Elizabeth stared at him horrified.

'Oh yes my dear and the prices they are paying now will cease and owners will accept what they are given.'

'But surely they can't force people to let them take their horses?'

'They can and they will should the need arise.'

'Not ours, surely, why only the farm, carriage and trap horses are broken to harness.'

'That makes no difference, the army needs quality horses for offi-cers and breaking some of the rest to harness will not be considered a problem. Very few, will be exempt.'

'But our horses are our stock, our living, Robert.'

'Then let's hope should the time come that you have friends in high places.' He studied his nails. 'I'm not without certain influence myself, Elizabeth.'

Crestfallen, Elizabeth considered his words. She knew if it should come to Robert's prediction their world would be in ruins.

Later, in the yard, as Robert made to take his departure, John strode across to him, his hand outstretched. 'Well Robert, the best of luck to you. Let's hope the powers that be are right when they tell us it will soon be over.'

'Yes. We've enough wrongs to right nearer to home without crossing the channel.' Robert's eyes swept over John before mounting his horse which one of the grooms had brought out. Nodding to Elizabeth, Robert rode out of the yard, leaving John only too aware that he had not taken the hand he had offered.

Elizabeth ran back into the house and spread the newspaper on the floor, kneeling over it she re-read the advertisement to which Robert had drawn her attention. Then glancing above, read another,

OHMS. Wanted Cavalry and light draft horses for Gunners from 15.2 to 16 hands high, age from 6 to 12 years and sound. Major A. W. Waite of Loughborough Road, West Bridgford, Nottingham will attend at Bradwell and Sons Horse Repository, King Edward Street, Nottingham, each day between the hours of 9 am. and 12 noon for the purpose of inspecting and purchasing horses. Owners of hunters are asked to get them up from grass, as horses of this class are urgently required.

Her mouth felt dry as she slowly folded the newspaper.

Shortly after noon that day, John and Elizabeth carried lunch up to Mary's room. It was not one of Mary's better days. A nurse, one of two, recently installed by John, adjusted the pillows and made her patient as comfortable as possible. Mary rewarded her with one of her sweet smiles. Elizabeth felt a lump rise in her throat, feeling the helplessness of seeing her mother's health deteriorating. A wicker table tray was carefully settled in front of Mary before the nurse left the family together. Elizabeth smiled encouragingly at her mother, seeing with dismay the minute portion of lunch before her.

'Come on Mama, eat up, cook will be overjoyed if you ask for a little more.'

'Darling, how optimistic you are, so full of life and enthusiasm, you're the best tonic I could have. Come and sit close by the bed and tell me what you've been doing this morning.'

Elizabeth put her tray on the bed and pulled her chair as close as she could get to her mother. 'I rode out first exercise, we went right round the windmill bridle path to Viawell and back by Moor Lane to give the horses some road work. Do you know Mama, autumn is coming prematurely this year with summer having being so hot and dry and as it was such a bright morning everything looked golden. I really think it's one of my favourite times of the year.'

'My dear, you say that about every season and what about winter when you compare hoar frost to fairyland, they're all your favourites, each season in turn. That's what being young is all about.' She reached out and stroked Elizabeth's head. 'Such beautiful hair, so dark and glossy, just like your Papa's hair was when I first met him. So handsome...' she smiled across at John, 'and still is.' She looked from one to the other, then back to Elizabeth. 'I pray my darling Elizabeth that you will meet someone like Papa, kind and handsome.'

'Perhaps it will be someone I already know Mama.'

John looked up from eating and glanced at Elizabeth but her expression gave nothing away.

'Maybe darling, you have a such a jolly crowd of young friends, I remember thinking so at the summer ball. It seems so long ago now, yet it isn't. It's quite frightening at the speed with which events have changed since then.'

John shook his head. 'You're right Mary, it doesn't seem possible that so much has happened in that time.'

Mary picked at her lunch. 'Our country at war, our young men leaving daily. Oh John doesn't it make you thank God we haven't a son to be sent away from us?'

John nodded. 'War, what does it achieve?' and without waiting for any answers or comments turned to Elizabeth and asked. 'Did you tell Mama of Robert Oakley's visit?'

'Not yet Papa,' Elizabeth glanced out of the window.

'Robert called?' Mary enquired.

'Yes Mama, he was in uniform, he called to say goodbye. He says that he'll be going away soon.'

Mary's forehead creased, 'What a worry for this family,' she said, adding, 'such a charming young man.'

VIII

It was some weeks later that Robert procured his first leave and could scarcely contain his irritation with his family. For days he had been haranguing them as to whether or not they would be going on their annual visit to Scotland to stay with Ralph's sister. Robert had promised his friends, old and new, a leave to remember and had no wish to disappoint them.

Eventually, his family decided to keep to their usual custom and it was with considerable relief that Robert saw his parents and sisters off to the station in Ralph's recently acquired Rolls Royce Silver Ghost driven by Vernon his father's chauffeur/gardener. It was due to Robert's express promise that he would not drive Ralph's precious Rolls himself during his father's absence, but, should the need arise, avail himself of Vernon's services, that Ralph reluctantly agreed for Robert to have any use of the vehicle.

Following their departure he set about making preparations, primarily taking stock of his father's cellars and urging Tomkins to organise the servants into provision for his guests. His family hadn't left it a day too soon, Robert thought, when, the following morning ignoring his promise to his father he drove the Rolls himself and sped through the village, causing to his satisfaction, a considerable stir. When he reached Nottingham Midland Station he scarcely had time to down a couple of glasses of whisky when the gathering of porters announced more succinctly than the timetable board, the imminent arrival of the train from St. Pancras. Sure enough, within minutes, the great steam engine pulled into the platform and leaning precariously out of a first class carriage window were three young men in uniform of about Robert's age.

He greeted them as they leapt from the still moving train. 'So, you old renegades, what have you been up to eh?' He tossed the nearest porter a florin instructing him to load the hide suitcases being pushed to the front of the guards van, into the motor car. After the usual ritual of back slapping and ribald comments the four made their way unerringly into the station buffet, renewing their acquaintanceship over innumerable Scotches.

'So, old chap, what are our plans then?' asked Jarvis Melton, winking broadly at a young girl clad in an overall, who giggled into the cloth she was using to wipe the table tops.

'Oh for God's sake Jarvis,' the Honourable William Berkley looked the girl up and down through the monocle he affected. Turning to Robert he grimaced and enquired. 'Has the town got much to offer then old boy?'

Robert waved a finger somewhat unsteadily. 'Wait until you see what I have arranged by way of company for supper. I've an excellent memory of your taste William and yours Jarvis,' then turning towards the third young man. 'Yours, Harold, I'm not so sure of.'

Harold Farnham looked aggrieved, 'I s... say Robert...'

The others laughed uproariously. William readjusted his eye glass and nudged Harold. 'Got to make a start somewhere, don't you know, nothing like a pretty gel to get a chap going eh?'

Harold laughed with them, protesting half heartedly. After finishing their drinks they made their way to the Rolls parked outside the station and now laden with cases.

'She's a beauty,' Jarvis enthused, climbing into the driving seat and examining the controls.

'Try her,' Robert invited, 'I'll direct you to Oakley, so long as we all get there in one piece,' he pulled a face at the others. 'I've planned a splendid evening for us all.'

'Can't wait old sport,' William told him as he climbed into the back seat. Robert started the whispering engine for Jarvis as the others whooped and whistled appreciatively, causing a few amused stares, then guided them through the town which was thronged with horse-drawn traffic, the odd motor vehicle and crowds of people. An air of optimism was apparent in the laughter and camaraderie coming from groups of young men in the uniform of one or another of the services. The raucous occupants of the Rolls headed towards the green horizon, west of the city.

The party, having lunched, bathed and changed, returned via the same route some hours later. Jarvis made a reasonable job of parking outside a fashionable hotel close to the Theatre Royal, where a liveried doorman opened the doors of the car for the four friends to alight. Scarcely had they done so before two porters were unloading overnight bags under his supervision. Once through the revolving doors and into the luxuriously panelled reception, it was apparent that Robert was not only expected but was a valued patron of the hotel. The first floor suite into which they were shown by the manager himself had numerous bedrooms leading off a large sitting room complete with bar, gramophone and white clothed dining table laid for eight.

The manager whispered obsequiously to Robert. 'The young ladies have already arrived Mr. Smith, shall I have them escorted up?'

Robert pulled out his watch. 'Give us a few minutes for heavens sake,' he said, irritability giving way to amusement as he reminded himself of the discretion of the place and the hotel policy that no ladies were allowed in any of the public rooms unless accompanied by a gentleman. Where, he wondered not for the first time, did the hotel 'accommodate' company invited to join guests there? He must remember to ask Sybil sometime. The man, to Robert's further amusement, made a half bow before leaving the room.

'I say M...Mr. Smith, you've got them all jumping here by Gad. I gather you're damn well known in the place,' Harold stammered, grinning.

Robert inclined towards a light from Jarvis and drew on a cigarette, then moved towards the bar and a large silver ice bucket packed with bottles of champagne. 'Damn right I have, after all I can soon transfer my business elsewhere should the need arise. Now come on, let's drink to the evening ahead.' He deftly uncorked the first of the bottles and poured the bubbling wine into four glasses, handing them around. 'To a pleasant interlude gentlemen between training and posting. May the evening come up to our expectations.'

'And to theirs...' William added raising his glass as there came a soft tap on the door. Robert admitted four attractive young women. The elder, a heavily made up sophisticated woman in her early thirties, kissed Robert on both cheeks, 'Sybil, my dear, good to see you, Robert greeted her. 'How are you?'

'Couldn't be better Ivan and you?'

Over the top of her head, Robert observed William raising an eyebrow at the second pseudonym, noting with admiration the speed at which William recovered himself and awaited the introductions.

'Sybil, may I introduce my friends. Gentlemen, Sybil and her friends. Sybil nodded graciously and beckoned a fair haired petit young woman with an hourglass figure, 'Lillian.'

The girl stepped forwards and nodded towards William, Jarvis and Harold, who was fiddling with a cuff link that had come adrift. She crossed the room to Harold and offered her assistance, coaxing the gold links through his cuff whilst he shifted his weight from one foot to the other, colour suffusing his cheeks.

'Elsie,' Sybil's voice again as a tall redhead of Junoesque proportions smiled warmly around the room.

'Gad, you're a fine looking gel.' The Honourable William adjusted his monocle, took her hand and led her to the champagne.

Sybil half whispered to Robert, 'Ivan dear, Marion sends her best love, but she couldn't come tonight, the poor darling's not well. But you know Marion, she would never let her friends down and asked her cousin who's staying with us to come in her place,' she looked a little anxious, 'I hope that's alright?'

Robert's face was bland as he looked at the fourth girl, introduced as Dora. Pretty, but brash, lacking the urbanity of the other girls he thought fleetingly. He paid her scant attention for she was soon whisked away by Jarvis whom he could have forecast would be taken by her blatant charms.

Soon the party was in full swing, Jarvis had the gramophone going and a few champagne bottles were already upside down in melting ice. The buffet supper did credit to the chef and they dined off creamed chicken vol-au-vents, cold sliced rare beef, honey roast ham, an enormous green salad and a citrus sorbet, followed by a good selection of cheeses and fresh fruit.

Robert had instructed that they were not to be disturbed, so when the food was finished with, he pushed the serving trolley out into the corridor and invited Sybil to dance. He found her interesting for many reasons, not least her business sense, knowing she ran a very discreet 'house' in the city, only introducing her girls to the best society. As they danced, Robert thought over the years of their liaison, secure in the knowledge that her interest in him was purely mercenary, she was not in the least offended should he ask for another companion, indeed she would go to some lengths to accommodate him to his satisfaction.

He smiled, an inward, rather unpleasant smile as he dwelt on their attempts at his satisfaction, their unconcealed shock at his humiliating and often painful demands, for all he was sure that Sybil had briefed them of his needs. No, Sybil was the pick of them, her timing was so accurate, his body began to stir as he thought of her tigerish attempts to defend herself before succumbing to his demands. He dug his nails into her back and pressed her tightly against him, he could feel perspiration beginning to break through her blouse, the heat of her body releasing waves of the earthy fragrance of musk with which he associated her and he felt a quiver of anticipation. He whispered into her ear and led her towards one of the adjacent rooms, his low laughter silenced by the door which he closed behind them.

William was swaying in a corner of the room with one arm around Elsie and the other around a bottle of champagne. From time to time Elsie broke free and danced provocatively around him, she had shed her jacket, and the high necked blouse of fine lawn she wore clung to her breasts which she showed off to advantage by raising her arms as she danced gypsy style and lowered them with a shake close to his face. William thrust the monocle into his pocket, dumped the champagne and picked her up, with a shout of, 'Gad, you're a fine figure of a gel,' and whilst she screamed with laughter, carried her clumsily into a private room.

Dora, a glass of champagne in her hand, was on Jarvis's knee, dizzy with wine and encouraging Jarvis's attentions. This was more like it she thought contentedly, just as her cousin Marion had promised. A young gentleman with plenty to spend on a girl - such good food and champagne. But even more than any of this, Dora hugged a new found knowledge to herself like a trophy, for the evening had already revealed more than she could have anticipated in her wildest dreams. Later, as she lay in Jarvis' arms in the luxuriously appointed bedroom, she had quite decided that this was the life for her and as her ambition soared, she thought with scorn of the local lads she knew and of their coarse talk and insensitive fumblings. All but one... her forehead creased into a frown for a moment but then she became aware of Jarvis' renewed caresses to which she responded avidly.

Lillian rose from the chaise longue where she and Harold had been sitting, she was a little at a loss to know how to handle the situation. She poured two glasses of champagne slowly, racking her brains for an answer then crossed the room to him holding the glasses before her. Harold reached for one as Lillian stumbled. The contents of both glasses poured down the front of her gown of green velvet.

'Oh Harold, my lovely gown, my favourite one, it's ruined.' She turned her attractive hazel eyes upon him. 'What can I do, please help me.'

'I s... say I'm awfully sorry Lillian, I don't know how it happened. Perhaps you should go into the bedroom and take it off and hand it to me, I'll see what the hotel staff can do with it.' He coughed. 'Err, if they can't do anything, I'll jolly well buy you a new one Lillian, that I promise.'

'Oh thank you Harold, you're such a kind person.' She disappeared into the bedroom but within seconds called softly to him. 'Harold dear, I can't get the gown off by myself, it's so difficult with the buttonholes wet with champagne.'

Behind the closed bedroom door, Harold battled with the buttons and conscientiously managed every one so that the gown fell away. Lillian looking sweetly into his uncertain face was at her most help-less, whilst subtly encouraging his hesitant caresses with well prac-ticed innocent acquiescence.

❧ ❧ ❧

'Bloody good night Robert, I salute you,' Jarvis shouted from the sad-dle, his voice carried away by the wind as the four friends thundered across the parkland behind the hall the following afternoon. He reined the bay hunter he was riding and turned to the others. 'Wicked little vixen mine turned out to be, I'm covered in love bites, looked a fine bloody spectacle in the bath I can tell you.'

'We'll take your word for it,' the Hon. William drawled. 'Sounds quite obscene.' He turned to Robert who had drawn alongside him, 'Did me proud old chap, woman to drool over, wouldn't mind seeing more of her... I'll rephrase that, having already seen a lot of her and what a lot there is to see, much I add, to my enormous pleasure. I mean, see her again don't you know.' He closed his eyes and shifted awkwardly. 'Gad, why are there occasions when a saddle is so bloody uncomfortable. I swear saddlers go out of their way to make sure there's not enough room behind the pommel, for a chap in an embar-rassing condition. Bloody malevolent lot, saddlers, thought so before. Do you know, out hunting last season, Mrs. Millington Owens dis-mounted in a spinney, presumably to answer a call of nature, natural-ly I averted my eyes as a gentleman would, yet when I looked back sometime later she went out of her way to tantalise a chap, fiddling about behind a froth of lace and showing off her superb legs. Had to negotiate a couple of jumps almost immediately after, thought I'd do myself an irreparable mischief.'

Robert and Jarvis laughed loudly at his revelation whilst Harold frowned, intent on scanning the horizon.

Jarvis shouted to Robert. 'What is your Sybil like then, you seemed to know her damned well, is she worth a bite?' He winked at the others. 'Just what are you keeping to yourself you old devil?'

Robert smiled slyly. 'She's not my Sybil, she's anyone's Sybil who can afford her and the value, I can assure you,' he rolled his eyes, 'is phenomenal. Whatever one's pleasure, a night with Sybil transports one into a sensuous paradise, experiencing everything a chap could visualise in his most erotic dreams and then a whole lot more. Take her on by all means, we'll all need some memories to carry into war and I doubt the most exclusive French whore you could find would be anything but a prospective student for Sybil.'

Jarvis rolled his eyes, then reached across and poked Harold with his whip. 'Go on, surprise us, tell us how you made out with the little blonde?'

Harold's face flushed. 'You really are bloody c... crude Jarvis, Lillian was sweet and needed coaxing. I wonder now if I took advantage of her, she lay so trustingly, b... but seemed to enjoy my attentions. I've always been a bit scared of girls you know, but this one left it all to me and I surprised myself by my ar... ardour.' He ran a finger around his collar and looked appealingly at the others. 'Do you think it was very wrong of me to, well, you know... she really was so innocent yet at the same time so agreeable, she totally bewitched me.' He smiled reflectively. 'Really it all happened because we spilt champagne down her gown and I helped her to undo it.'

The others roared with laughter.

'She's got your number,' Jarvis quipped. "Oh Harold, my stays are too tight, could you help loosen them?' or 'My chemise is cutting into my breasts, I hate to have to ask you...' A pretty blush and you're there. Well, good for her and for you, at last we're making something of you."

'You can be b... beastly, Jarvis,' Harold said, looking to the others for support.

'Nonsense my dear boy,' William smiled benignly. 'Finest gel you could have had, agree with Jarvis, she got your number straight away, thought so when she started fussing over your cuff link.'

Harold frowned and it was obvious to the others that he felt they hadn't understood the situation at all.

✂ ✂ ✂

Over pre-dinner drinks in the library the group revelled in a maudlin summary of the effects the war was having on their lives already. William's disclosure of a career was met with some astonishment.

'Damn it, I'd just succumbed at last to my father's demands to do something useful with myself. Got accepted onto the Board of a prestigious banking house in the City. Made a cracking good investment in the form of a property just off Park Lane.' William took a large pull from a glass of Ralph's excellent white Burgundy. 'My esteemed father thought my new responsible lifestyle would put me in good stead to propose to Miss Penelope Cuthbert Jones whom I met at her coming out. The Berkshire Cuthbert Jones don't you know. Now what's a chap to do eh? Jump in with both feet or see how the war goes. There's so much talk it will be all over by Christmas.'

Robert refilled their glasses. 'Let's drink to it, get over there, sort the bastards out and be home by Christmas to continue our lives.'

The Hon. William focused his monocle on Robert. 'You're a dark horse, Oakley, what of your civvy plans? We don't see much of you up at the smoke these days, surely there's no interesting fish to fry around here?'

Robert gave him a cynical smile. 'You'd be surprised William, I've my family continually urging me to propose to our neighbouring landowner's daughter, his only issue I might add. A tempting thought, for all her looks are a bit off putting, as the joining of our lands would make an estate of considerable proportion by the standards of any county.' He leaned back in the leather chair and reached for his glass, 'This possibility is the most likely one, but first I have my eye on a wild filly who I am determined to break. It's a challenge that both obsesses and excites me. There are so many ways to achieve one's desires, but I find the ideal opportunity inevitably arises, with a little help of course.' Robert sensed the unflinching gaze of the others and laughed.

'Don't you find new fruit all the sweeter for tearing it off the tree instead of waiting for it to fall? Virgins can be such bores. I suppose that's why so many of us find it necessary to find a variety of consolations when we are eventually lumbered with some simpering heiress.'

'God forbid,' Jarvis reached for the bottle. 'I'm almost glad I'm estranged at the moment from my old man. I tried to tell him there's a limit to how much hunting, shooting and fishing a chap can endure, or being in the bloody country for that matter. Threatened to cut off my allowance and all the usual penalties, so I took off and found myself a studio in Pimlico. I'd just acquired a most interesting following of artists and eccentrics when my old man stumps up for a commission for me and had me clapped into uniform. If he ups my allowance too I shall have no alternative but to become reconciled before leaving for France. Can't stand any more of Mater's tears though, got to say that. Bloody war. Still, probably be a lark.'

Harold who had been listening to the revelations of his host and guests, joined in. 'I suppose my life is comparatively dull compared to all of yours,' he said simply. 'I am, or at least I was, totally happy at home, helping run our estate before the outbreak of war. There is no interesting female in my life, nor can I think of anyone who would fit the bill around where we live, so I suppose all in all, my lifestyle seems a bore to the rest of you.'

'Nonsense my dear Harold,' William spoke kindly. 'You acquitted yourself very well last night with a young lady; let's hope that will stand you in good stead for others you will invariably meet, even in the course of your quieter lifestyle on the estate, though that's sadly changed now. Hey ho, the experience will be beneficial in any case, for when you meet girls now, you will approach them with a new found knowledge and confidence.'

Harold smiled thinly. 'Oh I wouldn't want Lillian to ever think that I'd used her for experience, she was so lovely.'

'They all are dear boy,' Jarvis laughed. '*Vive la difference.*'

'I'll drink to that,' the Honourable William pushed his monocle firmly into place and drained his glass.

During dinner that night, Tomkins moved close to Robert and coughed discreetly.

'What is it, Tomkins?'

'May I speak to you Mr. Robert?'

'What is it?'

Tomkins glanced significantly in the direction of the door. 'Perhaps if you could spare a moment Mr. Robert.'

Robert threw his napkin down, sighing heavily. 'Alright, alright, excuse me gentlemen.' Turning to Tomkins he indicated to a footman by the door. 'See that my guests are well attended to.'

'But of course sir.' Tomkins inclined his head towards the man and whispered instructions to him.

Once the door was closed behind him, Robert turned sharply to the butler. 'Well?'

'There's a... young woman here to see you Mr. Robert, she will not go away and threatens to make a scene if you refuse to see her.'

'Who is she?' Robert demanded.

Tomkins fielded the question, 'I took the liberty of showing her into the pargeted room, being the closest to the door,' he said meaningfully.

Robert grunted, curiosity overcoming his annoyance at having his meal interrupted.

Tomkins opened the door of the pargeted room for Robert to enter. A young woman stood in front of the huge empty fireplace with her back to him. Robert nodded for Tomkins to leave. As the door closed behind him the girl turned, though the low wattage electricity did nothing to identify her to him.

'Who are you and what are you here for?' he asked, tightening his lips in annoyance. 'Do you realise I have guests who have just sat down to dinner?'

The girl was nonplussed. 'To talk, Mr. Robert that's what,' she answered impertinently, 'and if you don't want everybody in this place to know what I've come for, you'll listen to what I've got to say without causing me to raise my voice.'

'How dare you speak to me that way,' Robert squared his shoulders. 'I ask you again, who the devil are you and what do you mean by coming here?'

'Amongst other things, to renew the acquaintance of... Mr Ivan Smith.' Uninvited, she took a seat on an oak settle by the side of the hearth, laid her hands in her lap and waited.

Robert felt the stirring of unease. Against his instinct, he crossed the room to the settle, taking care not to get too close to her and studied her face. He saw she was coarse and brash... brash, that was it, the girl who had stood in for Marion last night, the girl who had appealed to Jarvis. He looked at her with distaste, what the hell was she doing in his home?

As if reading his mind, she said, 'I bet you're wondering how I knew where to come?'

Robert's unease increased as she spoke again.

'Look hard at me Mr. Robert, you've known me all my life.'

'Rubbish, get on with your business before I have you thrown out.'

Her eyes narrowed. 'Oh I don't think you'll do that. If I tell my Dad about you and what your friend did to me against my wishes, he'll kill you both.'

'Against your wishes, from what I hear, you damned nearly ate him.'

'Been talking about me have you?'

'No, not at all.'

She gave a high pitched giggle. 'Well I don't care if it's your friend or you who pays me a hundred pounds to keep my mouth shut, because that's what it'll take.'

Robert stared at her. 'You can open your mouth to the world for all I'm interested, you'll get no hundred pounds from here.'

She began to button her coat. 'Right, you don't give me any choice, the next person to interrupt your dinner will be my Dad.'

'And who's he?'

'Frank Lupton, blacksmith and wheelwright to the estate.'

Robert paled, his father thought the world of Lupton. The family went back in Oakley almost as long as his own. The blacksmith was a giant, there was nothing he couldn't do with iron, God, the man had hands of iron, no one took liberties with Frank Lupton, anyone on the estate or in the village would verify that. Robert's mind was working at double speed, if he paid the girl this time there would be another and another time, if he didn't he could see Lupton breaking his head, neither prospect appealed to him. Damn, damn, damn, he cursed Sybil for bringing her, he cursed Marion for being ill but most of all he cursed the overconfident creature in front of him. Call her bluff, that's what he'd do. He faced her squarely. 'Tell me, is you father aware of the way you spend your nights?'

For the first time she faltered. 'He knows I'm staying with my cousin in Nottingham and that I do a bit of waiting on with her at the restaurant she works for sometimes. He must know we go out of an evening.'

Robert didn't miss the opportunity to exploit the crack in her veneer. 'I'm sure he'll know that, but does he know the rest, tell me that?'

'I can't help it if I'm asked out to a respectable supper and then taken advantage of can I?'

'Rubbish and I shall tell him so.'

The girl struck a pose and resorted to bravado. 'You'd better pay up Mr. Robert, I don't want to be stuck in Oakley for the rest of my life, I want more, and a hundred pounds from you will be a start. I might make a move on to certain other people around here as well, you'd be surprised what I know about some folk in this village.'

The girl was a hideous bore he thought, let her yattle on, maybe she would hang herself with her mouth. He half listened to her as she began to count on her fingers.

'I know your precious cook Mrs. Wain sends parcels of food from the hall kitchens, by the carrier, to her sister in Derbyshire. She wraps them in the clothes your Mam gives her. That Mrs. Oldham, your laundress, has Smedley one of the gardeners, in the laundry with her, romping on the sheets from the hall, before they're washed I hope, Mr. Robert.' She smiled nastily and continued counting. I know that hoity toity Miss Elizabeth O'Malley Sullivan is so obsessed by a stable lad that she can't keep her eyes or her hands off him. I know that the Parkins' killed a pig by...'

'You know what?' Robert had jolted as if by an electric current.

The girl began again, counting as she went. He let her talk, asking her to elaborate on each of her revelations. He feigned interest and then. 'How do you know about Miss O'Malley?'

'I've watched them, they ride out together early in the mornings, go off for hours sometimes. Touching, gazing at each other and rolling in the hay I shouldn't wonder. Makes me sick. He's got above himself. I went through village school with James Gretton, always did think he was above the rest of us.'

'Refused you behind the school ash pits did he?' Robert enquired coldly, feigning indifference and gathered from her expression that he had struck near the truth. He looked at her for a moment, 'I'll tell you what I'm prepared to do for the sake of my friend, I'm going to give you ten pounds.' He held up his hand as she began to protest, that's more than you're worth, perhaps some of your other information was worth more to me that your lying allegations regarding my friend. He took two large white five pound notes from the inside pocket of his dinner jacket and dropped them onto her lap. 'Now get out and don't come back or your father will know all about your nocturnal ventures. My friends and I are free agents, whilst you my dear are nothing but a slut.'

Robert did not go immediately back to his friends at the dinner table, instead he went to his room, where a small bedside lamp gave off a dull light. He caught his reflection in the mirror, dim and faceless and with one almighty blow of his fist, shattered the glass.

IX

Mary put her arms around John as he lifted her from the bed to carry her downstairs. His throat constricted at her frailty and he was agonisingly aware that she weighed less each day. He felt her breath on his cheek and the softness of her face against his neck as she laid her head on his shoulder. He was nostalgically conscious of the delicate fragrance of the floral toilet water she always used, which reminded him now as ever of their early days together, it seemed to him the essence of her serenity. He placed her gently in her favourite chair in the drawing room where she could look out onto the walled garden. As he settled her and spread a wool blanket over her legs she gave him a smile of incredible sweetness. His heart hurt with love for her, with compassion for her and with fearful apprehension for them both.

'Is there anything I can get for you?' he asked as he smoothed the cushion behind her head.

'No thank you, John darling,' Mary reached out her hand to him, stroking the side of his face as he bent over her. 'I shall look out into the garden, I have so many happy hours remembering how we all but lived out there, especially after Elizabeth was born and we would sit with her on a rug and watch her kick her legs and then learn to crawl and walk, she did it all in the garden didn't she?'

John smiled at the recollection. 'She was an outdoor baby, child and girl and is now an outdoor young woman who gets more beautiful every day, but how could she be anything else with such a beautiful mother?'

'My darling, we both know that Elizabeth is more like your mother than me.'

John smiled wryly. 'Well, certainly her colouring and I will admit, her ability with horses, yet many of her ways and indeed her kindness are your gift to her, just as you gave her the greatest gift of all, birth.'

'No, John, it's the other way round, our darling Elizabeth gave me rebirth, they thought I'd give up when she was born if you remember, but when I heard her cry I struggled so hard to come back from the journey I had set out upon, I couldn't bear to leave my darling baby and husband. God has been so good to me, I've had all these years with you both, years of wonderful happiness and fulfilment.' She pressed his hand to her cheek, 'I love you so much.'

John knelt beside her and buried his face in her hair, fearful that she might see the brightness of tears in his eyes, 'I love you too Mary, with all my heart. From the first time I saw you I knew I would love you forever.'

'Forever darling, that's a long time.'

'Not long enough,' John breathed into her hair.

❧ ❧ ❧

Elizabeth, James and a couple of the lads were industriously cleaning tack, a fire burned brightly in the grate of the large tack room.

'Phew, it's hot in 'ere,' Dick Hartley, the younger of the two observed, rubbing a grubby piece of towelling across his forehead.

'It has to be,' the other lad, Bill Myers told him. 'Heats the water, dries the serge backing on the saddles and harness and other tack, and airs the rugs an' all,' he waved a partly assembled bridle at rugs hanging to dry and at the high shelves where rows of rugs and dust sheets were tidily folded. The lads had been chatting as they worked for half of the afternoon to the amusement of Elizabeth and James who caught each other's glance from time to time and smiled indulgently.

'My brother's just joined up in a cavalry regiment, he says the army issue tack and harness is as hard as iron,' Dick said as he fastened the reins onto a supple double bridle.

'Poor horses, they'll be galled raw,' Bill answered with feeling.

'Aye and they're not the only ones either, my brother says the men are too. He says it's wicked.'

'It's wicked anyway, sending horses into war.'

'Well what's worse, he reckons they're going to send thousands more, thousands upon thousands,' Dick emphasised the point. 'They reckon there's horses tied up in the streets, lined up as far as a mile from the railway stations some days.'

'Where are they getting all them from?'

'What they can't buy they've started commandeering, stealing them some say, for what they give for them. Isn't that right Miss Elizabeth, what they're doing?'

Elizabeth sighed. 'It seems so Dick, we're hearing terrible stories. I heard the other day that the sister of a Duke had her favourite horse commandeered out of shafts. Surely they've enough horses by now. I was reading in the paper only yesterday that the French and Belgians have already sent practically all the suitable horses they've got for the war.'

'They won't take any from here will they?' Dick looked at Elizabeth. 'They won't will they Miss Elizabeth?'

Elizabeth bit her lip. 'Please God not,' she answered fervently, glancing at James, who spoke up firmly.

'Come on now, we've got a job to do and it'll be woe betide us if this place isn't ship-shape and Bristol fashion by the time Pa gets the feeding under way.'

Elizabeth looked at him gratefully. Her beloved James, she knew, shared her present anxiety and the helplessness she felt at seeing her mother failing a little more each day. Her thoughts turned to her father and to his total, selfless devotion to her mother. She stared into the fire, she knew now what such love could be between a man and a woman, for in these past weeks, she felt, if it were possible, that she loved James even more than ever for his strength and absolute dependability. She stifled a catch in her throat which was not lost on him, he looked into her eyes and closed his own for a second in complete understanding. Elizabeth swallowed hard, fighting tears, conscious that without him, she doubted she could hold up as she was doing for the sake of both her parents. During this agonising time she had learned to push the thoughts of any of the O'Malley horses being commandeered to the back of her mind, praying along with the rest of the country that the war would end quickly, though she acknowledged to herself with a shudder that there was no sign of it doing so.

The door of the tack room opened suddenly and the little group glanced up, expecting to see Tom, but it was John. His face was blanched and he looked across at his daughter.

'Come with me Elizabeth. Tom's gone to fetch Father Ryan and is calling on the way there to ask Doctor Morley if he'll come as quickly as possible.'

James, who had jumped to his feet, exchanged Elizabeth's glance briefly before she followed her father out of the stables. As they ran across the yard John spoke hurriedly, 'Mama took a turn for the worse whilst downstairs, we've got her safely back into bed but it's not good, not good at all.'

Elizabeth tore into the mud room, stripped off her work clothes and after washing and changing in precious seconds, joined her father at the bedside of her mother. Though barely conscious Mary opened her eyes and gave Elizabeth the sweetest of looks as her daughter took her hand. 'Mama, I do love you so.'

Mary formed the words so softly that it seemed to Elizabeth as though Mary's soul was speaking to her, 'I love you, my darling child.'

Elizabeth lay her face on the hand of her mother lest Mary would see her tears as they ran unchecked onto her mother's hand.

'Don't cry my darling, please don't be sad, we've known such happiness.'

From the opposite side of the bed John looked down upon the back of his daughter's head, her dark hair, which had come unfastened, was spread untidily across Mary's hand on the white counterpane. His eyes were blurred and try as he might, he could not dispel the mist before them through which he saw his wife and daughter. He became aware of Mary looking at him and fought for her sake, to regain his composure as their eyes met and a glance of absolute understanding passed between them.

Slowly, Mary closed her eyes and for a terrible moment he thought that she had slipped away without their priest reaching her in time. Elizabeth raised her head as John leaned over Mary and put his arms around her, drawing her to him as though his strength could flow into her and keep her with him. He felt her shallow breath near his ear and settled her gently back amongst the pillows. There was a soft tap at the bedroom door. Quietly he rose and to his relief, admitted Dr. Morley, who put his hand on the shoulder of his friend before they crossed the room to the still figure on the bed.

John put his face close to Mary's, 'Andrew's here to see you my darling, Elizabeth and I will wait outside. We'll only be outside the door,' he added, kissing her forehead.

Mary tried to smile, but didn't open her eyes. Reluctantly John and Elizabeth left the room whilst Doctor Morley examined his patient. He came out, folding his stethoscope and met John's eyes, shaking his head sadly. 'There's no more I can do John, her heart's failing. I'm so very sorry.'

John closed his eyes. 'Pray God Father Ryan gets here soon. Tom's taken the fastest trap pony.'

'I'll go downstairs and bring him straight up.'

'Thank you Andrew.'

John and Elizabeth returned to the bedside. John stroked Mary's forehead as he took her hand holding it to his cheek and murmured quietly to her.

From the bedside drawer, Elizabeth took a white cloth, two candlesticks and candles and a crucifix from the mantlepiece, assembling the little altar she regularly made by the bed for her mother when Father Ryan brought her Holy Communion, adding a small vessel of water and hand towel. Hot tears poured down her cheeks and she dare not turn towards the bed until she had fought to get them under control. Mumbling an excuse of fetching a fresh box of matches, she left the room and stood with her back to the door allowing the tears to stream unchecked for a while before drying her eyes and collecting the matches from the lamp cupboard on the landing. Voices came from the front door, silently she thanked God that Father Ryan had arrived as she returned to the bedroom with the news.

'Father's here Mama dear.'

John rose to meet the priest.

Elizabeth took the hand that John had laid on the counterpane. 'It will be alright Mama now Father Ryan's here.' She felt the softest of acknowledgement from Mary's hand.

Although not of their faith, Doctor Morley made a silent prayer of gratitude as the priest was admitted into the room of his patient and friend.

Father Ryan put his stole to his lips, then placing it around his neck spoke quietly to Mary turning his ear close to her to catch her frail whisper. John and Elizabeth knelt by her bedside and listened to the ancient words of absolution and in their grief watched her anointing.

Shortly before midnight, Mary died.

✤ ✤ ✤

Elizabeth sat in the window seat of her bedroom. It was, she reflected with sadness, four weeks since the terrible loss of her mother. She laid her head back on the folded shutters.

'Oh Mama,' she called to the silent room, 'how can I bear losing you?' She dashed tears from her eyes with the back of her hand. 'How can I comfort Papa when I can't bear it myself.'

Elizabeth closed her eyes and thought of her father. His grief was inconsolable. It was as though he had formed a shell around himself, making him singular and impenetrable. He spent much of his time at the hall with his old friend and antagonist, Ralph Oakley, leaving Tom to manage the yards and deal with much of the administration.

Elizabeth breakfasted alone. As was becoming his custom, her father did not appear until later in the day, very often, she knew he was sleeping off a heavy night's drinking with Ralph. She picked at the scrambled eggs and crispy bacon, sent in by cook, which Elizabeth knew was a kind endeavour to encourage her to eat.

The house reverberated at the sound of heavy bangs on the door knocker. Glad of an excuse to leave the table, Elizabeth dashed from the room and down the entrance hall, beating the parlour maid to the front door. Remembering herself she stood back whilst Jenna opened the door to two men. Elizabeth felt her knees weaken as foreboding stole through her. The elder of the two, a stout individual, untidily dressed in breeches, brown boots and a tweed jacket was the first to speak.

'We're here to see Mr. John O'Malley Sullivan. Is he at home?'

Elizabeth moved forwards. 'No. I'm his daughter, can I help you?'

From the top of the stairs, John's head appeared over the banister as his voice boomed down. 'What the hell's going on? Thought the house was being knocked down.'

'There are two men to see you Papa, I didn't think you were at home.'

The men glanced at each other after apparently observing John's dishevelled appearance and dressing gown. Again the elder spoke producing a tattered card from an inside pocket, 'Cornelius Leverett,' he introduced himself. Then indicating to the other man, introduced him, 'Mr. Oswald Watson, Veterinary Surgeon to the War Office.'

He raised his voice up the stair well. 'We are authorised buyers of horses necessary for the war effort.'

John paled. 'Show these gentlemen into the office Elizabeth, I'll be down directly.' He disappeared from the banister.

'If you'll please wait here for a moment.' Elizabeth turned and dashed into the office off the hall. There she scanned the tidy room for any sign of their business lying about, she saw none, for Tom and herself had been meticulous in their paperwork and filing. Slowly Elizabeth turned and made her way back to the entrance hall and the two men waiting there as her father joined them and led them into the office himself.

'If you'll be so good as to make a brief inventory of your stock Sir,' Leverett began.

John looked askance at the man. 'My stock, you say. The work of generations, I say.'

'Yes, yes sir, but this is war and circumstances alter all that.'

The vet endeavoured to placate John and said in an even voice. 'If you could co-operate with us Mr. O'Malley Sullivan it will save us all time. We've got other calls to make.'

John lifted his pen, it felt as though it weighed a hundredweight. He closed his eyes for a moment comforting himself that they couldn't take his breeding mares now heavy in foal, or the three and four-year-olds in the process of being broken in and schooled, or, thank God, his stallions. Then there were the youngsters in the care of Bob Sherwin up on his Derbyshire land, they too would be safe by virtue of their ages. Wearily he opened his eyes, pulled a sheet of paper from a desk drawer and began to write.

Elizabeth fled to Tom and Annie's cottage, where she burst in, interrupting the family's breakfast. Tom and James leapt to their feet.

'My God, Elizabeth what is it?' Tom began to choke on a piece of toast. Annie patted his back, whilst James got him a glass of water.

Tom recovered himself as Elizabeth shouted incoherently. 'They've come to commandeer our horses. They're here now, talking to Papa.' She clutched Tom's arm pulling at him. 'Please come quickly, let's take the horse's away that they'll be interested in. James, let's lame them, a stone wedged in the foot, anything to prevent them from being taken. You hear of all kinds of things people try to prevent them from being commandeered.' She was sobbing between her words. 'There'll be the hunters, the carriage horses, the Welsh cob, you don't think they'll consider taking the three and four-year-olds do you? Dear, dear God, what are we to do?' She wrung her hands as Tom and James grabbed their coats and pulled on their boots. Annie wrung her hands as, helplessly, she watched them dash out together.

They found the middle yard in a flurry of activity. Elizabeth saw to her dismay that all of the lads had been pressed into helping show the horses the men were interested in. She watched in horror as the carriage horses were being trotted up and down, along with the Welsh cob. There had been no time to implement any of her desperate plans. From the bottom yard Minette along with the other hunters were being led up for inspection. Lads carrying headstalls seemed to be everywhere.

Elizabeth rushed to her father's side, 'Papa, stop them, they can't do this. They can't come into our yards and take what they like.' Her voice trailed off miserably as she studied her father's face.

'They can and they will Elizabeth, and we can't do a damned thing about it, they're doing it everywhere. We must just be thankful that your mother didn't see this day.'

James clenched and unclenched his fists as the vet had the entires led out. He turned to Tom, 'Surely Pa, they won't take stallions. Whatever are they thinking of?'

His question was answered by a rough looking individual who appeared to be the spokesman of a band of men that Leverett and the vet had left in the yard whilst they had conducted their business with John in the house.

'They wants 'em for officers, they like a spirited mount, can't get enough of this sort. Same as these four-year-olds, just what they're looking for.'

The last of James' hopes died quietly. He watched in anguish as Elizabeth dashed from one group of horses and men to another then back to her father and over to Tom and himself.

'Tom,' she called wildly. 'There must be something we can do. I know, ride up to the hall quickly and see if Robert Oakley is still there, he'll help I'm sure he will. He's already told me that he's not without influence.'

Leverett forestalled him. 'There's no horse leaving this yard Miss until we've completed our business. There's no point in making a fuss, we're within our rights to be here and do what we have to. Don't you realise the county's at war? Patriotic gentlemen have been sending their hunters since August and getting good prices. Them 'us have their horses commandeered will have to take what they're offered now and lump it.'

Elizabeth caught Tom's eye and inclined her head in the direction of the hall, nodding meaningfully. Tom backed away from the group as Leverett continued his remonstrances, saying loud enough for John to hear. 'You must have seen the papers, we've been standing at Bradwell's Horse Repository in Nottingham for months buying horses for the War Office. As I say, patriotic gentlemen were the first to offer theirs.' He glanced slyly at John, 'Irish connections haven't you, sir?'

'What's that supposed to mean?' John retorted angrily.

Leverett sniggered. 'No offence meant I'm sure. Nobody's got a better eye for a horse than the Irish.' He jerked his head at the lad leading Rua. 'Take him to the vet.'

Elizabeth rushed to Leverett and put her hand on his arm. 'No, please not that one, I beg of you.'

John stepped forwards, for a moment Elizabeth thought he was going to attack the man. 'That young stallion is only four-years-old.'

'And exceptional if I might say so and if your records are correct, like the others, he's rising five.'

'Where's the sense in taking the entires? We've thirty brood mares.'

'Ah,' the man turned. 'That's something we must talk about. The War Office are putting a ban on breeding for the duration. The mares must be allowed to go barren as reserve stock for the military.'

'But that's preposterous,' John spluttered the words in fury and disbelief. 'What then, pray? What's to happen to our bloodlines?'

'Thoroughbred stock, yes, hunter stock, no.' He hit the side of his boot with his stick. 'Anything suitable between the ages of five and twelve years.'

'I thought it was six and twelve?' John retorted.

'You seem very aware of our requirements, sir, so it should interest you to know that buying is ultimately left to our discretion.' He laughed dryly. 'We'll no doubt be taking any age soon.'

Tom returned to the stud, his face was flushed and sweat ran down the sides of his temples. He wove his way through the throng in the yard to John and Elizabeth. 'It's no good John, Captain Oakley's not on leave and the squire's at a shoot over at Viawell.'

John nodded slowly, then turned and made for the house. A pile of five pound notes left by Leverett, toppled and fell from the low wall of the yard as Elizabeth, Tom, James and their lads watched help-lessly whilst the veterinary surgeon, with a brand hotted up on the tack room fire, burnt an arrow on the hooves of the commandeered horses and had them put into War Office headstalls. They were led away, four to a man with the exception of the entires, which were led ahead, one to a man.

Out of ninety-two horses at the stud on that day, thirty-nine were commandeered. Sixteen hunters, including Minette, twelve four-year-olds, three entires, including Rua, four carriage horses, three of the eight farm horses and the Welsh Cob. The prices John had to accept, against their peace time value, ranged between one fifth and one quarter of their worth.

Frantically, Elizabeth sought her father, but found he had locked himself in his dressing room and was deaf to her supplications. She walked slowly from the house and made her way to Tom and Annie's cottage.

In the village pub, Leverett raised a foaming glass of beer to Watson who stared unhappily at the tap room floor. 'What a haul eh? Here's health to young Captain Oakley.'

X

On her fifth visit to the hall in two days, Elizabeth finally found Robert at home. Tomkins had her shown into the morning room where Robert was finishing an early breakfast alone.

He rose to greet her. 'Good morning Elizabeth, how very nice to see you. Have you breakfasted?' He indicated the sideboard bearing numerous covered dishes.

'Yes, yes, Robert,' she rushed towards him and hurled herself into a chair he had drawn out for her by his side at the table. 'I've already called several times but you were away.'

'My dear, I am away most of the time now, being responsible for supplies takes me all over the country.'

She scarcely listened to him, words tumbling from her. 'Have you heard? The very worst has happened, many of our horses have been commandeered including our stallions,' she wrung her hands. 'We're facing ruin.'

Robert reached for her hand, 'I was home very late last night, father told me something of this. Come, my dear. Tell me calmly.'

Elizabeth forced herself to take several deep breaths and then launched into an account of the happenings two days before. When she had finished, Robert took her other hand and looked into her eyes which were brimming with tears.

'Elizabeth, how absolutely awful. God, how I feel for you. Did they really take the stallion you had such high hopes for?'

Elizabeth nodded miserably, 'James and I have worked with him for the past four years. Please, Robert, get him back for us, we've become so close to him.'

Robert didn't move a muscle, 'I'm sure you have, my dear.'

If the intonation in Robert's voice had changed at all, Elizabeth was unaware of it. She stared down at his long white hands which held hers. 'You told me, not so long ago, that you're not without influence, Robert. Did you mean it?'

'Of course I did Elizabeth and without putting too fine a point on it, being in supplies is not without advantages. Believe me I shall do everything in my power to find out where they have taken your stock and use those advantages on your behalf.' He looked above her head, 'I was of the opinion that the War Office were still buying all the horses they need from those willing to make the sacrifice.' Again the inflection in his voice was lost on her. He laid her hands on her knees and rose, crossing the room, where he rang the bell by the marble fireplace. He had scarcely resumed his seat when there was a tap at the door followed by the appearance of Tomkins.

'Yes, sir.'

'Bring fresh tea and an extra cup for Miss Elizabeth.'

When the door had closed on Tomkins, Robert turned back to her giving her his most enigmatic smile. 'You say you could face ruin Elizabeth, let's be realistic now, I'm sure you'll leave here feeling a little better if we can talk of this from a business perspective.' He spread his hands depreciatingly, 'I've no wish to pry into your family business, you understand, but how exactly could the commandeering of some thirty-nine horses out of, what, over a hundred, counting young stock, be the ruin of you?'

'We've been forbidden to breed the mares until further notice Robert, insanity isn't it? Apparently mares have to be kept in reserve for this awful war. After the next crop of foals at the beginning of the year they have to be left barren...' Her voice caught as fresh tears spilled down her cheeks. 'You know what that can mean. It's not always easy to get mares in foal again when they miss a year, or more if this terrible war goes on.' She endeavoured to control herself as the tea arrived, aware of Tomkins' discreet glances from one to the other.

'Is there anything else I can get for you sir?'

'No,' Robert snapped at the man.

Despite Elizabeth's distress, she found herself squirming at his treatment of the butler whom she had always found to be kind and helpful. She made an effort to give Tomkins a faint smile.

Robert stirred his tea and without looking up, asked, 'How is your father taking all of this?'

Elizabeth stared at the carpet, eventually she answered with resignation. 'To be honest, Robert, Papa hasn't been well since mama died. I really don't know what we would have done without Tom and James, they're such a strength.' She stood up suddenly. 'In fact, I must get back, we're terribly short handed, two more of our lads have joined up.'

He rose languidly. 'You must, my dear, we can't have Tom and James put out can we?' His sarcasm was wasted on her.

She looked into his eyes. 'Promise me Robert, that you will get at least some of our horses back, please...' The pupils of her eyes, dilated with tears seemed almost black. In contrast, Robert's pale eyes hardly differed from the whites.

'Trust me, my dear. You are one of my oldest and dearest friends, good heavens, we've known each other from childhood. It wouldn't be honest of me to feign modesty at such a critical time regarding the extent of the influence I do have. You will have to trust me.' He put his hands on her shoulders and leaned forward to kiss her cheek. 'I'll keep you in touch with my progress, try not to worry now that you've put the matter into my hands.'

She suffered his kiss absently. 'Thank you Robert, you don't know what this means to us.'

After Elizabeth had left, Robert remained in the morning room and helped himself to a second breakfast, heaping his plate with bacon, kidneys and eggs. He found it difficult not to laugh aloud and contented himself with a contemptuous smile as he recalled Elizabeth's words.

'Please Robert,' how she had grovelled. Just the beginning Miss O'Malley, better than he had hoped for. His body stirred pleasurably, no pulling away from him this time as there had been at the ball. 'Trust me, Elizabeth.' He was on the verge of giving way to laughter when an angry shadow crossed his face, 'Tom and James.' He could see again the softening of her features when she had mentioned that accursed upstart, and the words of the blacksmith's slatternly daughter came back to him. By God he would make them suffer, no one crossed him. He felt the blood rush to his head and he clenched his fists, he'd make them pay. Tipping off Leverett had only been the beginning.

Elizabeth strode out towards home across the parkland, the shortest distance between the hall and the stud. For the first time in two days, she felt some hope in her heart. She began to run, eager to repeat Robert's promises. John was still in his dressing room when Elizabeth raced up the stairs, she called to him from the door of his bedroom, then burst in surrounded by fresh morning air.

'Papa, you'll never guess. I've finally found Robert at home and he's going to get our horses back, or at least some of them. What do you think of that?'

John continued to fasten the buttons of his shirt, 'Elizabeth my dear, that's a vain hope. I've already spoken to Ralph as you asked me to on this very subject and he made it quite clear that neither Robert nor anyone else can interfere with the War Office.'

Elizabeth twisted a cord which held back the window drapes. 'But Papa, Robert is in a unique position. He's responsible for supplies now and has all kinds of influence. He's told me this himself so I know he'll be able to work something out.'

John sighed. 'Darling, please don't be too hopeful. I'm sure Robert means well and is trying to help you cope with this blow, but try not to count on anything.' He held out his arms to Elizabeth and held her to him.

She lay her head on his chest. 'We must keep hopeful Papa. I know Robert is our only chance and I'm putting my trust in him as he asked me to.'

'He asked you that did he?'

'Yes Papa, and I told him that he has my trust. Robert will help us, you see.'

John stroked Elizabeth's hair as he had done so often when she was a child, then lay his cheek on top of her head and stared across the room at a photograph of Mary.

✿ ✿ ✿

Elizabeth found James alone in the feed room sorting and tidying shelves. The familiar smell of grains and molasses met her.

'James, I've been to the hall, spoken to Robert about him getting our horses back.' She closed her eyes. 'Thank God he's going to get straight onto it.'

A frown crossed James' face. 'You've been asking favours of him, whatever do you think he can do about the horses now they've gone?'

'Oh James, don't you start. Papa has just said that, but you're both wrong. Robert has influence, he told me that some weeks ago when he mentioned commandeering. He's our only hope. I stressed Rua, we must have Rua back. He's our future.'

James' frown deepened, 'Robert Oakley had already spoken to you about commandeering? When?'

'The day he came in uniform, to see me, you remember?'

'Who raised the subject?'

'I can't remember, does it matter?'

'It could do Beth,' he said slowly.

Before he could speak again, she put her hands each side of his face and looked into his eyes. 'James, darling, don't you see, he's the one person who can help us. He has rank and influence. The reason he hasn't been sent to France yet is because his command is dealing with supplies, supplies of every kind and he is in control. Don't you understand that's how he can do something, wheels within wheels as they say. Who better to work on our behalf than Robert? Had he been at home when those awful men came, he could have prevented the commandeering, I just know he could. He's actually said this morning that he thought the War Office are being offered all the horses they need. I think they jumped the gun coming here and I think Robert does too.'

James lifted her hands from his face whilst Elizabeth continued to stare into his eyes, he felt her willing him to agree with her, instead he found himself seething with rage and despair.

'Robert Oakley is a rotter. He would no more help you than he would fly. You should never trust a man like him. Why some of the lads who've recently left had been talking amongst themselves and none of them could understand why horses have been commandeered from here first. There's been no commandeering so far around these parts except here. They think that the War Office buyers were tipped off. Who would do that Beth, ask yourself?'

'No one would do that. We've no enemies, Papa is always fair in business. For goodness sake, we guarantee our horses. No, James, they're mistaken, no one would do such a thing, not buyers and certainly not neighbours. I will not believe that.'

'Won't you now? But then who's talking about buyers or neighbours. More like someone with influence and position.'

She stared at him. 'Who?'

James held her gaze.

Elizabeth's eyes opened wide. 'You can't be implying that Robert... Surely that's not what you're suggesting? I know he can be arrogant, but not downright wicked.'

James turned his back on her and resumed work, stacking mineral blocks on the shelves.

Elizabeth spoke in a low clear voice. 'You'll never make me believe that of Robert.' She stared at the back of his head. 'He asked me to trust him and that's what I intend to do.'

He spun around. She reached out to him, but he shook her off angrily.

'You little fool,' James threw himself down onto a corn bin and ran his fingers through his hair. 'You're playing into his hands, just as he wants you to do.'

Elizabeth stood in silence for a moment in disbelief and then said, 'Don't speak to me like that.'

'I see, it's Miss Elizabeth now is it? Half an hour at the hall with

Robert Oakley changes things does it?'

She recoiled as if he had slapped her. 'Why are you being so horrible now we have a chance of getting our horses back? Robert's given us hope, don't you understand, something to cling to instead of the awful hopelessness of the past two days. I would have thought that you of all people would be pleased. Imagine getting Rua back.' She tried again, 'James, please tell me you understand what I've tried to do in asking for Robert's help. Don't make me feel that you're distancing yourself from me.'

'I might as well if you're going to turn to a man like him.'

'James, you're being ridiculous... and unreasonable... and so discouraging.' Her eyes filled with tears. 'I went to the hall early this morning feeling that it was all hopeless. I found Robert at home at last and he gave me his word that he will do his utmost. I know he will, he was so sincere and genuinely concerned for us.'

'Rubbish.'

'I don't have to stay to hear you talking like this. Why can't you put your trust in him as I have done and keep faith with him?'

They stared at each other momentarily and then she turned and dashed out of the building. James watched her go, his emotions conflicting. Half of him grieved for her, the other half feared.

※ ※ ※

John's lethargy filtered down to everyone at the O'Malley Stud.

'He's a changed man,' Tom confided to Annie, 'I didn't think things could get any worse after the tragedy of losing his beloved wife, God rest her, but now...' He sucked hard on his pipe. 'I suppose it was understandable how he neglected the paperwork after Mary's death, but Elizabeth, me and James were just about keeping on top of it for him, but since the commandeering everything's in disarray, records, bloodlines. Elizabeth's written to buyers, cancelling orders for horses which have been commandeered. It makes me so damned mad Annie, if what happened here is happening all over the country, well to some, not all I should think, not them whose faces fit. Makes you wonder how they got onto this stud so soon doesn't it? And what of taking horses below the specified age?'

❧ ❧ ❧

John looked across the library in the hall through a haze of cigar smoke and alcohol. He was fully aware that he'd had far too much to drink though his mind hadn't yet snapped, thereby blocking out the memories he fought to keep at bay.

'Come on old friend, let me help you to bed, stay over here tonight, give us an earlier start for the shoot in the morning,' Ralph cajoled.

'Later,' John lay his head back into the corner of the leather wing chair in which he was sprawled. 'You go, leave me here for another half hour.'

His tone didn't invite dissension and Ralph laid his hand for a moment on John's shoulder. 'As you wish John, but don't make it too late.' As he left the room he looked pointedly at Robert who was pouring himself a brandy. For a while the two men sat each side of the fire without speaking. Robert broke the silence.

'How is Elizabeth?' he enquired pleasantly.

'Well, though devastated about the commandeering.'

'I hope she's taken heart that I'm doing my best on that front.'

'Yes, Robert, damned good of you, she has indeed taken heart.' John's eyes were closed and even when he raised his glass to his lips, he didn't open them.

'You're a lucky man to have such a charming and spirited daughter, sir.'

'I am Robert.'

'There's none in these parts to rival her beauty and character. I hope I can justify her faith in me.'

'I hope so too Robert.'

Robert studied him from under his lids, then slowly and deliberately crossed over and filled John's glass to the brim, returning to his chair and continuing to watch the older man take steady pulls at the brandy. As John slumped lower in the chair, Robert made his move.

'How about a last game of cards?' he enquired.

'No, I think not.' John slurred the words.

'What a blessing for your family that my forebear wasn't so mean a sport.'

'Robert, I've told you before what they were like in those days, there was nothing to pick between them.'

'Has all the mettle been bred out of the O'Malley's nowadays, have they no sense of sportsmanship left in them...'

The words hung between them. John took the bait. Struggling to get out of the chair he leaned forwards somewhat unsteadily towards Robert. 'For God's sake, get the cards out and let's settle this issue, which seems to be festering within you, once and for all.'

✄ ✄ ✄

The two men faced each other across a card table. John arranged his hand through the mist before his eyes. A strange unreal feeling stole through him and for a moment he felt almost as though he were his grandfather, back in time, holding the hand which was to win him, outright, the Oakley farm which now formed their stud. He raised his eyes to Robert, searching the arrogant young face for a clue to the hand he held, but all he gained was a confident stare. Again, he felt the liaison with his grandfather, this time with fleeting caution, but dispelled it with the confidence of inebriation. John looked at his cards, a king, a queen, ten of hearts, eight of spades, six of spades. He stared at them. Hearts, the suit of love, spades, the suit of death. As he spread the cards on the green baize, he wondered what the hand had been which had helped to make their fortune.

Robert was in no hurry to show his cards. His pale eyes swept over John for long enough to cause discomfort in the elder man. With an amused twist of his narrow mouth, he then laid his hand before John. 'As we agreed, best of five.'

John glanced down and closed his eyes with a groan, God in his mercy, what had he been thinking of? The hand was imprinted on his closed eyelids. Two aces, a king, nine of hearts and five of clubs. He felt the blood rush to his temples as Robert sauntered over to his father's desk and returned with a chit and quill.

'If you please sir.' He stood, poised above John.

Filled with fatalistic horror at what he had done, John took the pen and paper and signed away his home, land and holding in Oakley.

❧ ❧ ❧

'How dare you take advantage of a bereaved man who had drunk too much? God Almighty, hasn't he endured enough these last weeks?'

The veins in Ralph's temples stood out against the purple hue of his face as he poured disgust and contempt upon his son the following morning.

'You strutting young cock sir, you're no son of mine. Where is this so called debt of honour you forced him to sign?'

Robert raised one eyebrow and surveyed his father with cool indifference. 'On its way to my solicitor, father.'

'I'll send someone down to retrieve it this very minute,' Ralph tugged at the bell pull by the fireplace.

'I said my solicitor father, I did not say yours.'

'What, you've taken it upon yourself to attempt to change our legal advisor, you overstep yourself sir.'

'No, father, I have no business with your solicitor.'

'Well wherever it is, get it back, go now.'

'I doubt they will have received it yet.'

Ralph rubbed his forehead wearily. 'Get down there yourself now, Robert, and sort out this ghastly mess, mistake, call it what you will to them but retrieve the paper. I will not have a man I call my friend treated in this manner by you or anyone else.'

Robert lit a cigarette and surveyed his father through the smoke, 'I don't choose to do so.'

Ralph strode across the room as if to strike him, stopping within inches and peering into the face of his son. Robert didn't flinch, neither did his expression lose its cool contempt. In contrast Ralph face became even darker in fury.

'How dare you, sir, how dare you?' Ralph repeated the words in disbelief.

'You're doing yourself no good father,' Robert exhaled smoke as he spoke. 'You will bring on your apoplexy allowing yourself to over-react in this way. The man put up his estate and lost it to me. It's as simple as that. As simple as his family procured it in the first place.' He studied his nails. 'Do you think our ancestor whined for the debt to be overlooked? No, of course not and neither will he. He gambled his land freely and of his own choosing. There's no more to be said.'

'You're so right, there is no more to be said, the whole issue is void and I intend breakfasting now with John and telling him so. Whilst we are out shooting you can do as I say and get down to this new solicitor fellow and do something about this absurd paper.'

Robert stubbed out his half smoked cigarette and with an ill concealed smirk, walked out of the room.

      ✄ ✄ ✄

John stayed on after the shoot, drinking with Ralph. Mid-afternoon, though it was raining heavily, he staggered off towards home in the direction of the park, game bag over his shoulder, gun broken across his arm. From the east door of the hall, Ralph saw him off, his eyes troubled with pain for his old friend. He waited until John disappeared over the horizon, sighed deeply and returned to the house.

The sun was getting low in the winter sky as John dumped his bag and gun and climbed the iron fence into one of the coverts, an enclosure like many on Ralph's land, crowded with glossy leafed evergreen rhododendrons. He sank down heavily in the wet foliage and lit a cigarette, a habit he had developed since Mary's death. He shivered and tried to swallow, but his mouth felt dry and dehydrated. He rubbed his face, massaging the muscles of his cheeks which bore the peculiar stiffness he recognised as one of the effects of too much alcohol.

Yet, strangely, his mind felt startlingly clear. If only that clarity had been there the previous night, he squirmed at the recollection. God in Heaven, what had he been thinking of? How could he face Elizabeth? How was he to tell her after she had lost her dear mother, then many of their horses including the red stallion, that he had thrown away their home and land so needlessly. What had been Robert's real intentions? All John could find in his favour was his interest in Elizabeth, maybe that was why he had been so determined to acquire her home. For all his faults, he was the son of his best friend, surely he couldn't be all bad, no one, John thought, was all bad. Robert wouldn't rob Elizabeth he decided, so maybe that was the way of it.

He thought of Ralph's kind words at breakfast. 'Just a young man's idea of a joke, John, don't even give it another thought.'

John knew that was not the case, but he trusted Ralph implicitly. Ralph would see it through, see fair play, he could rely on that.

He had never felt so low, he began to sob, rocking himself backwards and forwards in the knowledge that the bereavement he had suffered, the helplessness of commandeering and his own foolishness, were more than he could bear. He raised the cigarette to his lips, his hand shaking and inhaled deeply as he sought refuge in his memories whilst the sobs caught in his throat. The dear face of Mary filled his mind as he recalled the first time he ever saw her. She had been with a party of young people at the next table to his at the Wolds Hunt ball.

He remembered the exact date, the seventeenth of December, 1895. A date that had changed his life forever. He had fallen in love with her before she knew of his existence. He recalled how she had been laughing, yet, for all her amusement, he saw in her, a tranquil luminosity such as he had never encountered in anyone before... or since. It had been like a miracle, he thought, when following his determination to obtain an introduction to her, he had learned she was Catholic, indeed, from an old English Catholic family who had kept the faith through penal times.

He pulled a dead branch from behind him and settled more deeply into a hollow as he drew on his memories of their wedding day. He sensed again the atmosphere in the comparatively new Cathedral of St. Barnabas in Nottingham, hearing the swell of the organ reverberating through the magnificent Pugin building. He smelt the elusive fragrance of incense and saw the myriad of candles he had lit for her at the statue of the Holy Mother for whom she was named. John felt his eyes fill as he remembered turning to his bride as she arrived on the arm of her father, his first unbelievable impression of her in her wedding gown was as vivid now as then, that she was like an angel from heaven. An angel from heaven... He knew he would never have behaved as he had done with her beside him. John rested his head on his hands and wept for the love he could not live without.

He decided a gate would be the place, that was it, climbing a gate was the answer, the obvious place for an accident. John swung over the iron fence and picking up his bag and gun walked down the hill to the gate of Elm Copse.

Ralph was cleaning his guns when he heard the shot. An appalling premonition struck him. He called the dogs as he stuck his feet clumsily into muddy boots, grabbed his jacket and rushed out of the house, following the direction John had taken less than an hour before. The retrievers, Captain and Draper ran on ahead, noses to the ground and followed a straight line to one of the coverts. Ralph felt his stomach churn as he saw them check briefly before leaping through the rails and pursuing a trail downhill in the direction of Elm Copse. Before Ralph saw the crumpled body of his friend, the dogs had reached the gate and were giving tongue, howling their message of death.

Ralph walked towards them and dropped to his knees, then took off his jacket and covered his old friend from the onslaught of rain and soulful stares of the watching dogs.

XI

Elizabeth stood by the open grave. It was barely two months since it had been opened for her mother. She felt completely numb. An unreal aura surrounded her, as though it was all happening to someone else, to some poor soul who doubted that life could hand out any more grief. In the strange world into which she had taken refuge, Elizabeth pitied that soul for the heavy burden it carried.

Father Ryan read the words of interment as he sprinkled the coffin with holy water. Then the undertakers lowered her father's remains into the ground and offered her a vessel containing earth. Mechanically she took a handful, not even, she thought, the earth of Oakley which he had loved, but alien earth from a nearby town cemetery where a small plot was set aside for Catholics. Her eyes filled as she condemned herself, why, oh why, hadn't she brought a container of earth from his beloved Oakley? He must have done for her Mama, Papa had been a sentimentalist who would have thought of such things. O God, why hadn't she thought?

Aunt Martha, her mother's elder sister and now Elizabeth's guardian, took her arm and guided her to see the flowers which were present in abundance. Mechanically, Elizabeth looked at them and in the same way, kissed and shook hands with many of the mourners who, for various reasons were not able to return to the house for refreshments.

Although Tom and James had done their best with some of the three-year-olds which they had broken to harness since the commandeering, the animals were still green to drive and pranced about in the shafts. Elizabeth didn't appear to notice. Following the carriage were the traps, transporting the house staff, stable workers and in most cases, their families also. In happier times, many of these travelled together to St. Mary's, Hyson Green for Mass on Sundays and Holy days. The tragic procession was joined by other followers and wove through the small town east of Nottingham and uphill towards Oakley.

James and Saxon stood by Elizabeth as she stared listlessly around the room, whilst her Aunt Martha and her Irish relatives, Dermot, Finn and Daniel Sullivan hosted the reception. The sad gathering passed off almost without her feeling that she was part of it. Only when Saxon put his arm across her shoulders as his family left, did she feel the wetness of tears on her face.

The majority of the mourners eventually departed, leaving Elizabeth's relatives, Tom, Annie, James, various employees and Mr. Neeson the family solicitor, in the drawing room. Mr. Neeson fetched his briefcase from John's office. When he returned, he spoke gently to Elizabeth.

'My dear, it must seem to you to be a most inappropriate time to discuss business matters, but sadly it is my unfortunate duty to make known your late father's wishes.' Elizabeth sitting close to her aunt, turned her eyes to him without interest.

'With the exception of legacies to relatives, Tom Sharkey and various members of the staff,' here he mentioned their names, 'you are of course the main beneficiary. The two estates, the stud farm here at Oakley and the farm at Gatthorpe in Derbyshire, all live and dead stock, investments and capital, to be incorporated into a trust for you until you reach twenty-one years of age.' He smiled kindly at Elizabeth before continuing. 'Your late father nominated me to administer the trust, to meet your needs and advise you, and Tom Sharkey is to manage the business for you.'

�֍ ✤ ✤

Once back at the cottage, Annie put the kettle on and sat at the kitchen table in her funeral black. Tom and James who had followed her in, seated themselves opposite.

'I'll have plenty on Annie,' Tom said after a while of silence.

'You'll do as you've always done Tom, your best. That's why John entrusted Elizabeth's interests to you in running the business for her.'

Tom rubbed a hand over his face. 'Run the business - some hopes of that as we've known it. Now they're onto the stud they'll not leave us in peace. John knew that. He'd begun negotiations with his family in Ireland about the possibility of getting the brood mares over there before they foal so they can be served in Ireland and also the three-year-olds from here.'

'What will they do with them over there?' James asked him.

'Sell so many, keeping records of where any of the mares have gone to. That way we could eventually get some of the bloodlines back. Elizabeth, you, and me, need to talk about the horses we've got and make decisions of what we can consider selling. The remainder, which we must keep to a minimum, will stay at the Sullivan place in County Kildare. Mr. Neeson will arrange for their keep and expenses. We've none of us any idea how long this war will last but as John had begun to realise, we must make provisions. To leave the brood mares here would be a disaster, both for their breeding programme and the possibility of commandeering, and the youngsters we hope to send are getting older all the time and could risk the same fate.'

Annie got up to make the tea. 'How do you think Elizabeth will cope with all of this?'

'I'd like to think we could get her involved as soon as possible while Dermot's here, but with the terrible losses she's suffered you can see she's in deep shock. God help her.' They were quiet for a while. Annie sighed and began to pour the tea.

Tom stirred his cup, 'John was also talking about developing the arable side of the place when the horses are off it, get more hay from what's grazed now and plough some to extend our crops of oats. He planned on selling fodder to the military. They're shipping out mountains of it to France. Also we could produce good crops of roots to sell locally.'

'You do what John intended then, I'm sure Elizabeth will want to be involved as soon as she's able. It's a blessing Martha's staying with her.'

'Aye and Dermot too, he's offered to remain whilst we sort the horses out. He'll help us to get what we can shipped out of here. He's arranged with his brothers Finn and Daniel, to cope with their family business while he's away, they'll have plenty on too by all accounts.'

'Do they have a very big stud?' James asked him.

'Not a big stud, they breed a few horses like a lot of the Irish do, but they are mainly bloodstock agents. They're in quite a big way over there. You should see their place; it's like heaven on earth, close by the Curragh, green as far as the eye can see. I've loved it when I've been with John buying and selling.'

'Did your parents come from that part of Ireland, Pa?' James asked him.

'No, both sides were from County Cork. They came with their families as children in the famine, settled east of Nottingham close to each other and eventually married. My Pa worked with Shires, he loved the breed.'

They lapsed into their own thoughts. James was the first to speak again, returning to their earlier conversation, 'I didn't realise Mr. O'Malley had been up to making plans like these you've told us about, not since the terrible loss of Elizabeth's mother, I mean.'

'Since the commandeering James. I know he spent more time up at the hall, but he also spent time with his solicitors and with me. There were days when we had some good talks, so I know which way his plans lay, both in his hopes to avoid further commandeering in the future and also trying to compensate for the loss of business.' Tom sighed heavily. 'I'm sure he was thinking of getting his plans under way when he had the accident. What a tragedy, it would have helped him cope if he only he'd lived to become absorbed in these plans.'

Annie rose to refill their cups, 'I can't understand him having an accident with a gun, there was nobody more safety conscious than John. The others nodded.

James staring at the opposite wall said. 'It was almost as if there was more to it, something we don't know about.'

'He'd got enough that we do know about, his mind was just not on what he was doing in my opinion.' Tom looked down at the kitchen floor lest James would see his eyes watering. 'Before God, he was the best man I ever knew or will again.'

XII

It was a quiet time in the yards, everyone but Elizabeth and James having gone for lunch. In the seclusion of the loft, Elizabeth lay with her head in James' lap.

'I've an idea I want to talk to you about,' he told her.

'What is it?' she asked lazily, as she stroked his face and outlined the dimple in his chin with her fingers.

He raised her up and kissed her mouth tenderly with a gentleness devoid of passion then held her close to him. Elizabeth, her head pressed to his chest, heard the resonance of his words as he spoke again.

'When everything's sorted out with the horses, I'm going to get a job at the shell factory at Chilwell. Jobs are still being advertised, despite the large numbers being drafted there which include many of the injured from the war.'

She pulled away and faced him as she began to protest, but he silenced her.

'Hear me out Beth, there's not the work here to merit another person. With so many of the lads joining up at least it's saved having to let them go. Pa and the two elderly farm workers Joe Bingley, Eddie Smart and the remaining lads can carry out your Pa's plans to grow fodder for the army. I can change my job. I'll do it for us, they say there's good money to be earned and I could hold my head up more if I was earning independently of here.'

'I don't like to think of you working at a place like that. It's dangerous, apart from being confined indoors all day which you would hate.'

'Everybody's having to compromise nowadays, don't you see Beth? I'll work all hours, save hard, then we can begin to think of the future.'

'Darling James, you're all the future I ever want.'

'And you mine, that's why I want to do this, I've given it a lot of thought.' His voice was serious, 'I've nothing to offer you, that's what I'm trying to say.' His grey eyes were intense as he fixed his gaze upon her.

'You mean money? I have money, Mr. Neeson is going to see to it until I'm twenty-one and then Papa's arranged for me to take over, so it's not something that could possibly come between us.'

'That's not the way I want it sweetheart. It's you I want, not what you've got. We must wait for a year or two. When I'm twenty-one, Ma and Pa have told me that there's a little money coming to me from my parents, so with that and what I shall have earned, I should feel better about things.'

Elizabeth was silent for a while, then asked, 'Will I still see you every day if you take on this work?'

'Bound to, it's different shifts you know.'

'I don't like the sound of it at all.'

'Listen to me Beth, I've turned things over and over in my mind and I think I've hit on the ideal answer, also I can help out here when I'm not working, that's the advantage of shift work. I'll get the best of both worlds, don't you see?' He caressed her cheek with the back of his fingers.

She snuggled into his lap and closed her eyes. For the first time since her father's death, she was beginning to look ahead. 'If only I need never be any further away from you than this, my darling James,' she said quietly.

For some time James studied her sleeping form. For all of her spirit, she seemed so defenceless, curled up, head nestled in his lap. He noticed a delicate sheen on her closed eyelids as he lifted a strand of hair from her face and in the open neck of her shirt he could see his medallion of St James. He felt a great surge of love for her and a powerful longing to care for her.

❧ ❧ ❧

Although the amount of riding work was considerably reduced there were still the three-year-olds to be exercised and schooled and Elizabeth continued her routine of having breakfast between the first and second lots. Dermot, as he had promised had stayed on, and along with Aunt Martha had fallen into the habit of breakfasting with Elizabeth and discussing the progress which was being made with John's plans to date. The following morning after James' talk with her, Elizabeth received a formal letter from a firm of solicitors in Nottingham.

'It'll be from your Papa's solicitors m'dear, no more than a formality,' Dermot told her fondly as he left the table and crossed the hall to John's study, returning with a paper knife.

Elizabeth turned the letter about. 'They're not our solicitors and I don't recognise the names, Snide, Wilcox and Snide,' she frowned as she twisted off the seals and opened the envelope. The letter was brief and to the point, requesting that she attend their office in Beastmarket Hill, Nottingham, mid-morning two days ahead. She looked from one to the other and offered the letter to Dermot, 'I don't know anything about this firm.' Elizabeth shivered involuntarily. 'There's something about it I don't like. I would sooner speak to the older Mr Neeson, who has always handled our business.'

Dermot passed the letter to Aunt Martha catching her eye and raising his eyebrows before turning back to Elizabeth, 'I think you're right m'darlin' he told her, 'I'll accompany you and our first call will be on Mr. Neeson, we'll get there early before his appointments, sure and it's a pity we don't know the purpose of this.'

'What do you think it's all about?' James asked Elizabeth later in the day as they walked the fields checking the mares before dusk.

'I can't imagine, unless Papa had some private business with this firm,' her spirits lightened. 'It couldn't be anything else, could it?'

'You're right,' he acceded. 'Don't worry about it, you'll know soon enough.'

⚔ ⚔ ⚔

In his office, some two days later, Ernest Neeson could not enlighten Elizabeth regarding any connection with the other firm of solicitors, but neither Elizabeth nor Dermot could miss his disdain at their name. 'Best thing, keep the appointment and call on me afterwards,' he glanced at his diary. 'How about lunch? Ideal,' he offered his hand as he saw them out.

Elizabeth pulled on her gloves and linked her arm through that of Dermot as they made their way down The Poultry, past the Town Hall and across the market place to Beastmarket Hill. The impression Elizabeth formed of the premises of Snide, Wilcox and Snide inspired none of the confidence of the ones which they had just left. This, she felt, added to a sense of foreboding as they were ushered into the office of the senior partner. Mr. Snide, rose to exchange introductions with them and introduced his son, the younger partner. Elizabeth and Dermot were then asked to be seated, facing the two men across a large desk.

Mr. Snide senior seemed to Elizabeth to find the wall a foot above their heads more interesting than the people he faced. After clearing his throat, he formed a pyramid with his two forefingers. 'Did your late father confide in you at all Miss O'Malley Sullivan regarding any business he had with our client Captain Robert Oakley?'

'Robert? Why no. What kind of business?' Then for a moment her face shone with hope. 'You mean getting some of our horses back from the war department? Robert is working on that for us.' She studied the face of the man opposite but was disappointed to find no confirmation there. 'Is that it?' she added less optimistically, finding her answer in his lack of response.

Mr. Snide continued to stare above Elizabeth's head. 'The evening before your father's unfortunate er... accident, a game of cards took place at Oakley Hall between your father and Captain Oakley.'

Elizabeth swallowed hard, dear God what was coming. She felt the room had taken on an oppressive atmosphere, the air heavy and still, causing her to breathe shallowly whilst foreboding stole through her.

The man continued unremittingly. 'Your father put up his entire holding at Oakley and I regret to have to inform you that he lost his stake.'

The silence which followed his statement was merciless. Elizabeth lay her head back and would have fallen from the chair if Dermot hadn't caught her.

'There darlin' girl, bear up, let's hear this ridiculous story through.' He glared at the two men. 'What are you thinking of?' he demanded. 'Causing such distress to a girl little more than a child who has suffered two bereavements in as many months. Do you think she's not had enough without being affronted by this ridiculous story?'

Making no effort to reply, Mr. Snide took a paper from his desk and passed it across to Dermot, looking at them both for the first time. As his eyes slid across Elizabeth she saw how colourless and cold they were, an indication, she was convinced, of the man's character. Dermot took the paper and studied it. Watching him, Elizabeth saw hope die in his expression. In a voice, scarcely above a whisper, she said, 'Tell me.'

He handed the paper to her and stood behind her, his hands on her shoulders.

'This is your father's signature is it not?' The man behind the desk pursued his relentless task.

'Yes, it looks like it is.'

'And do you understand the meaning of this I.O.U. your father gave to Captain Oakley immediately after the game?'

'No, I don't understand, I don't understand at all. Why would my father throw away what we have, it's just not like him. He loved our home and the stud farm, he would never throw it away. I don't believe any of it.' She covered her face with her hands and leaned back on Dermot.

'Did you see your father on the day of the tragedy or the night before?'

'No, he stayed over at the hall, he did so on occasions since Mama died, he and the squire were very good friends and there was a shoot arranged for the following morning.'

'Did you see him at all before the shoot?

'No, I've already told you I didn't.' Her voice caught as she added quietly, 'I last saw Papa when he left for dinner at the hall early the previous evening.'

'So you could not have known of the fateful game?'

'No, and I don't believe it ever took place.'

Dermot tightened his grip on her shoulders and addressed Snide, 'Before any more is said, I advise Miss O'Malley Sullivan to consult the family solicitor. It's already arranged we see him upon leaving here. I would like him to see the I.O.U. as soon as possible.'

Snide retreated again behind the pyramid of his fingers before speaking. 'By all means, but it cannot leave this office. Now we have seen Miss O'Malley Sullivan, my office will contact him. He will of course, need to see the document before handing over the deeds to the property and I assure you Mr. Sullivan that everything is in order for the immediate transfer of the property which was won fairly and squarely by young Captain Oakley. Unusual, this day and age, but not unknown and I believe that the property has exchanged hands in this manner on a previous occasion?'

The man bared his teeth in a fleeting parody of a smile and it was all Dermot could do to control his impulse to strike him.

✼ ✼ ✼

Elizabeth could barely contain herself on the journey home, never, she acknowledged, would she drive horses beyond their endurance but her frustration with horses not fully trained to pulling the carriage caused her to bite her lips and pray for speed. Once the driver made to turn into the gates of the stud, she hung out of the window and shouted to him, to stay on the road.

'Child what are you doing?'

'I'm going to the hall, Dermot.'

'Mr. Neeson advised against contact with Captain Oakley at this stage, you must give him time to look into the legality of the claim.'

'I very much doubt he'll be there, but I'm going on the off chance.'

Dermot sank back into his seat. 'Alright, but let me handle it. Hear me darlin'?' Slowly she nodded as Dermot routed the driver to the hall.

Tomkins admitted Elizabeth and Dermot with his usual aplomb and evident regard for Elizabeth.

'Is the squire at home?' Dermot asked perfunctorily, his face sombre.

The butler, if curious, showed no sign of it. 'I'll go and see sir, please will you wait in the drawing room?'

Within minutes Ralph appeared and took Elizabeth's hands warmly. 'What a treat it is to see you my dear.'

He shook hands with Dermot. 'What can I get for you? A whiskey? I have Jameson's,' he added hospitably.

'Nothing sir, we have business we must discuss with your son.'

'With Robert?' Ralph frowned. 'Please sit down Elizabeth, Mr. Sullivan. If it's about restoring any of the commandeered horses to you, I crave your indulgence. Robert couldn't have done so. It was a foolish and thoughtless act on my son's part to give hope to Elizabeth, though I'm sure he did it with the best of intentions.'

Dermot paced the room. 'That is not why we're here sir; I've tried to convince Elizabeth that particular cause is without hope. With the tragedies she's suffered recently and the loss of many of her horses, I wouldn't have thought things could be any worse.' He stopped in front of Ralph. 'Things have become worse, infinitely worse and your son sir, is the cause of it. We've just learned that he tricked my cousin into some stupid card game whilst he was not himself. It appears your son won the game and demanded my cousin honour his stake, the family home and holding in Oakley.'

'How can you know of this?' Ralph was visibly shocked.

'Because we were summoned to the office of some tin pot solicitor in Nottingham this morning and told bluntly that Elizabeth's home now belongs to your son.'

Ralph passed a hand wearily across his eyes, 'I can't believe it, the whole matter was folly and I have insisted it be treated as such.' He turned to Elizabeth. 'My dear, you can't believe it is anything else. When I first learned of the affair I dismissed it completely, just an act of folly...' Ralph repeated, taking a rasping breath, 'I have already spoken to Robert, I absolutely forbade him to take anything so ridiculous seriously and as far as I'm concerned the whole sorry affair is over and done with. My son is in no doubt about this whatsoever. Madness, all of it. John didn't know what he was doing, no one, least of all my own son should have taken advantage of a man in the state that John was in.'

Clumsily he put his hand on Elizabeth's shoulder, 'I'm grieved my dear that you've had to learn of this at all. I can't comprehend what's in Robert's mind, but I will, by Jove, I will. He has yet another of his two day passes the day after tomorrow, though I fear this time it could well be embarkation leave.' He shook his head sadly. 'We can't have him leaving for France with this abysmal situation unresolved.' Ralph paused to force an unhappy smile at Elizabeth and pat her hand, then taking another searching breath tried to reassure her. 'We must resolve it and I'm sure we shall.'

ॐ ॐ ॐ

'I can't take any of it in,' James ran his fingers distractedly through his hair. Elizabeth stared into the embers of the tack room fire, seeing in the ashes a pageant of the day's events which she had just related to James.

'Surely Beth, when you all face him in a couple of days he'll be under pressure from every direction to let the whole thing go?' James knew that his voice was unconvincing, the premonition of evil which he had always had regarding Robert Oakley was engulfing him, he felt as though he was falling into an abyss, Elizabeth before him and he was reaching out to her whilst not quite being able to grasp her, save her, retrieve her from the hell into which Robert Oakley had thrown her. His loathing of the man made him feel physically sick, his stomach churned and his head pounded as the magnitude of the situation seized him. He took her face in his hands seeing her appalling panic at the enormity of her loss.

'Why James, why on earth would he want to do this to anyone, least of all me? I've done him no harm, I love his family as if we are related and they've always been so good to me. Please James darling, tell me why?'

James bit his lip and shaking his head averted his eyes, determined not to reveal his dismay.

She leaned her head on his shoulder and took his hand, tracing her finger across the palm. 'Do you know James, I would do anything, anything in the world to keep this place.'

☙ ☙ ☙

Elizabeth and Dermot faced Robert in the presence of his father two days later. The comparison between the two men was shocking to Elizabeth. Ralph, distress evident in his face which was dark red almost purple, mopped his forehead with a handkerchief, whilst Robert was pale, composed and supercilious.

Ralph was the first to speak. 'Now then sir, let's clear this up and be done with the matter. Tell Elizabeth and her cousin that the whole absurd business of this card game was just a stupid act of folly and that you intend to treat it as such.'

Robert lowered himself into a chair and rested his head against the upholstery, he took out a cigarette and lit it, calmly and deliberately, exhaling smoke, a half smile playing about his lips. Ralph, evidently misinterpreting Robert's manner, relaxed a little and invited Dermot to join Elizabeth on the couch as he himself sank heavily into a chair beside Robert.

'There now Robert, I'll say again, let's talk this through and have done with it.'

Robert picked a flake of tobacco from his tongue and examined it. 'There's nothing to discuss father, as I have already told you, Mr. O'Malley Sullivan showed no hesitation in putting up his Oakley farm, therefore sir, I have no hesitation in taking what I won in an honest game. My solicitor has the necessary legal proof and all I am waiting for now are the deeds.'

Dermot leapt to his feet. 'You young swine, you aren't going to get away with this.' He made to swing at Robert but was hampered by the bulk of Ralph as he lumbered to his feet and struck his son full in the face. Ralph reeled back clutching his chest and fell heavily against Dermot who broke his fall and lowered Ralph to the ground. Ralph was gasping for breath, his eyes bulging with effort and fear as Dermot loosed his collar and stroked his forehead.

'Ring for help Elizabeth.' He turned to Robert, 'As for you...' He shook his head and spoke through clenched teeth. 'Does your father have medicine?'

Robert studied his nails, 'I really couldn't tell you, my mother will know.'

'Well for God's sake, do something. Get up off your arse and find her, and fetch the doctor, you shouldn't need me to tell you that.'

Languidly Robert unfurled himself from the chair and with a disparaging look at the inert form of his father, sauntered from the room, passing Tomkins who, assessing the scene hurried over to a drawer in a *bureau plat* and produced a vial of tablets which he passed to Dermot.

Elizabeth, her eyes wide with horror and compassion knelt beside Ralph stroking his hands, then obeying Dermot's jerk of the head, left the room returning seconds later with Lenora, who rushed to her husband. Elizabeth, hardly knowing where she was going, wandered out of the hall by the door nearest to the stables and leaned against the door jamb covering her face with her hands as she took great sobbing breaths of air.

'No need for hysteria Elizabeth my dear, what is he to you?' Robert reined a bay hunter in front of her.

'Just go Robert, fetch Dr. Morley. Hurry.'

'Not so fast my dear Elizabeth,' he dismounted and stood uncomfortably close to her, his breath stale in her face. She twisted away from him and he grabbed her collar to turn her, tearing the fabric of her blouse away from her neck.

'What have we here?' he clutched the medallion.

A look of horror crossed her face. 'Don't you dare touch that, even you would not desecrate the image of St James.' She tried to retrieve it from his grasp.

'St James is it? James eh? A love token from the upstart?' He sneered, 'From one papist to another.' The icy penetration of his eyes sought her denial and when none was forthcoming an expression of uncontrollable rage replaced it and he tugged sharply, breaking the links and thrusting chain and medallion into the pocket of his jacket.

Elizabeth clutched at him. 'Give it back to me Robert, it's very precious to me.'

His mouth twisted into a travesty of a smile. 'Is it my dear? How very quaint.' His face hardened, Elizabeth watching, thought it took the appearance of an evil mask. She closed her eyes against the sight and moved her head from him in evident disgust. He struck the side of her face violently with the back of his hand. 'Don't dare turn from me whilst you're whoring yourself with that creature. You'll dance to my tune from now on, count on it.' He thrust her from him, mounted and was gone, gravel thrown high and into her face by the retreating hooves.

✄ ✄ ✄

From the time Elizabeth and Dermot had left that morning, James had been restless, he had worked hard at his jobs and then busied himself by the gates, casting anxious glances up the village in the direction of the hall where he expected to see the carriage returning at any moment. He heard the drumming of hooves of a single horse before Robert Oakley came into sight and watched as he thundered towards him.

Robert had passed the stud gates when he reined the hunter fierce-ly, the unnecessary force on the curb-bit causing the animal to roll its eyes and open its mouth in pain. He'd do his business with this swine now he thought, sooner than later, the old man could wait and be damned. It was his own bloody fault, after all if he hadn't endeavoured to humiliate him in front of the O'Malley clan, the old fool wouldn't have brought this on himself. He turned the horse and rode back to the gates, James stood upright, trowel in one hand and a stray sod of grass in the other.

'Open the gates damn you,' Robert barked at him.

James pulled the huge gates open and Robert rode into the yard, almost riding James down as he did so.

He reached into his waistcoat pocket and pulled out a half sovereign. 'Here lad, catch.'

Dispassionately, James watched the gold coin fly through the air towards him and fall at his feet.

'Pick it up.'

James gave him a look of disgust and made to turn away.

'Too bloody proud are you? Then perhaps you'll catch this, you bastard.' He reached into the pocket of his jacket, pulled out the medallion he had so recently torn from Elizabeth's neck and threw it high in the air towards James. An arc of silver glinted above him as James dropped the trowel and reached out, catching it.

'She was helpless with laughter when she asked me to drop this off,' he told James. 'I've never seen Elizabeth so amused.' His laughter echoed around the silent yard as he turned his horse and galloped down the lane. James stood until the hoof beats could be heard no more then made his way slowly to the cottage.

※ ※ ※

It was dark before Dermot thought of returning to the stud. He had sent the carriage home, not knowing how long they would be needed at the hall. Ralph had been conveyed to bed and made comfortable. Doctor Morley had left and upon Lenora's reassurance Dermot prepared to take his leave.

'Where is Elizabeth?' he asked, as they descended the stairs.

'I would imagine she is with our daughters,' Lenora answered, 'probably in the blue drawing room.'

But she was not, neither girl having seen anything of her and after a preliminary search Dermot accepted Lenora's offer of a trap, assuming that Elizabeth had returned home alone. He found this was not so and an all night search was instigated, Elizabeth being found at first light by a farm hand several miles from Oakley, wandering in a semi-dazed state, her clothing saturated and torn, her hands and face scratched by brambles, a large bruise on her cheek. She had been conveyed to the hall. A fever had already taken hold of her and for the second time in twenty four hours Doctor Morley was summoned.

✄ ✄ ✄

Elizabeth lay in a fever for almost a week. Lenora had a team of nurses installed, whilst she and her daughters fussed around the invalids. Martha had visited the hall daily, Dermot when he was able, due to his involvement with the horses. Both had been advised by Dr Morley only to sit quietly beside Elizabeth and this they had done.

By the end of the week she was strong enough to talk to them and learned that events at the stud had not moved at so slow a pace. Many of the brood mares had already reached Ireland and travel arrangements were in hand for the rest, with the addition of the three-year-olds. She was told that the remaining stable workers, were taking groups of horses to the nearby Kelingleigh station and accompanying them on their journey to Ireland, to be met off the boats by the younger Sullivan brothers and grooms. In their capacity as bloodstock dealers she knew that her relations anticipated no difficulty in selling any of the well reputed O'Malley horses, though in listening to Dermot, she sensed that it lay heavily upon them to have to do so. She was incredulous to realize that the only horses which would remain at the stud were five of the Shires which had been spared to them for the increased arable farm work and the trap ponies.

By the tenth day Elizabeth rose and dressed, her summons from the bell in her room was answered not by a servant but by Lenora herself.

'My dear child, what are you doing up, you know that Dr Morley left instructions for you to remain in bed for at least another week.'

Elizabeth kissed her cheek. 'How kind you are,' she said, facing Lenora, 'but I can't impose any longer on your hospitality.' She took the elder woman's hands into her own. 'You do understand Mrs. Oakley?'

'Please Elizabeth, how can we be so formal when I've nursed you as I would one of my own children. Of course I understand your wish to return home.'

A cloud crossed Elizabeth's face which was entirely lost on Lenora. 'What of Robert?' her hand moved involuntarily to her cheek. 'He's not here is he?'

'No, Elizabeth, sadly Robert was posted to France the day you took ill. He left strict instructions that you were to be well looked after, also... he left something for you.' She nodded her head conspiringly, misinterpreting the panic in Elizabeth's eyes. 'He was terribly anxious about you my dear.'

Elizabeth turned away saying, 'What has happened to my home, has he claimed it?'

'Oh Elizabeth, I'm sure Robert has only the best of intentions towards you. Do you know I think he has some long term idea that will be to your advantage. He's awfully fond of you, he told me himself that he has plans for you. Now what about that?'

Elizabeth felt as though cold water was being poured down her back and ignoring the question asked her own, 'I would like to look in on the squire before I leave. When will it be convenient?'

'I'll pop in and see dear, Ralph will be so pleased to see you.' She hesitated. 'You do know that his speech has been affected and he can't move his left side at all since he collapsed?'

'No I didn't, but thank you for warning me.'

Lenora left the room and Elizabeth collected together her belongings which Aunt Martha had brought.

After a short time Lenora rustled back into the room. 'He'll see you now Elizabeth dear, follow me, but for heaven's sake don't try to overdo things, for both your sakes, you know what Dr Morley has said.'

Elizabeth was shocked by Ralph's appearance but showed no trace of it. She smiled and took the right hand which Ralph offered. He tried to speak but the effort caused him obvious distress, exacerbating the high colour which had not subsided. After a short time Elizabeth kissed his forehead and took her leave, Ralph's eyes followed her as she left the room grieved to see his mouth still working in an effort to communicate with her.

Lenora made Elizabeth comfortable in the drawing room to await the carriage to take her home, disappearing for a moment and returning with a flat dark blue box which she gave to Elizabeth along with an envelope. Making an excuse to see if the carriage had been brought round, she left the room again as Elizabeth tore open the envelope. It was a letter from Robert. She shivered slightly and braced herself to read it.

'My dear Elizabeth, I plead your forgiveness for my unpardonable conduct on that terrible day when my father took ill. I can think of nothing but the appalling hurt I gave you both physically and mentally, it was all so out of character for me. I am truly mortified and beg you to understand that I was not myself seeing my father so near, as I believed, to death. You of all people may understand and show me the compassion of which I know you are capable.

'At the summer ball you looked so beautiful in blue, yet had nothing at your neck. Since then I have combed London to find this necklace which I hope you will accept with grace and forgiveness.'

Elizabeth opened the box which bore the name of an eminent Bond Street jeweller. The necklace was exquisite. The centre stone a large sapphire with graduated sapphires each side, all surrounded by diamonds set in platinum. She closed the box, leaving it on the table and began to weep for the medallion he had taken from her.

❧ ❧ ❧

As the Oakley carriage pulled into the top yard of the O'Malley stud, Elizabeth was overcome by a wretched feeling of loss, seeing the closed stable doors in the now silent yard. Only the presence of Aunt Martha and Dermot and their solicitous care in getting her indoors, temporarily eased the increasing anxiety, which had now settled upon her. She was horrified by her own weakness but fought to put a brave face on her return home.

Mrs. Bailey herself, bustled around, setting up tea on a small table by the fire in the drawing room and placing a poppy seed cake close to Elizabeth.

Elizabeth smiled at her. 'Thank you Mrs. Bailey, my favourite.'

Mrs. Bailey's eyes were bright as she attempted to smile. 'We've lost Jenna you see Miss Elizabeth, silly girl has taken herself off to work at the munitions factory at Chilwell. A lot are going there.'

Elizabeth paused for a moment, hearing over again her beloved James' plans to work at Chilwell. She must see him. She ate her cake obediently like a child and drank her tea. 'I'm going to Tom's,' she told them when she had finished.

Aunt Martha and Dermot exchanged glances above her head.

'No, mavourneen, I think not, you're not up to that yet.'

'Please Dermot, I promise I won't be long.'

He shrugged and put his hand up to Martha. 'Let her go. Only minutes mind, promise me?'

Elizabeth nodded. She made her way slowly to the mud room and collected a warm jacket, her legs felt as though they didn't belong to her and she stumbled through the postern door, almost falling into the yard. The dogs greeted her fondly and she stroked their heads in passing.

❧ ❧ ❧

At the cottage, Elizabeth knocked and heard the scrape of a chair and the clack of the latch being lifted as the door was opened. Her eyes met those of Tom as he admitted her and closed the door softly behind her. Annie was ironing at the kitchen table, a shirt which Elizabeth recognised as one of James', the heat of the flat iron releasing the smell of soap with which she was so familiar. She ached to see him, it had seemed so long.

As Annie acknowledged her, Elizabeth was shocked by her appearance, noting her red eyes and hollow cheeks.

'Where's James?' Elizabeth looked from one to the other. 'Where is he?'

Tom crossed the room and put his arm across Annie's shoulders. 'James enlisted the day you went to the hall, Elizabeth.'

Elizabeth felt the room spin around her as she sank to the ground.

PART THREE

WAR

Exiled afar from youth and happy love,
If Death should ravish my fond spirit hence
I have no doubt but, like a homing dove,
It would return to its dear residence,
And through a thousand stars find out the road
Back into earthly flesh that was its love abode.

Alan Seegeer, *Resurgam*

VIII

1914

South-east of Nottingham, Colwick Hall, stables and park, along with the race-course and it buildings, had been utilised by the regiment. In one of the four huts hastily erected in the grounds, James unbound the khaki puttees from his calves. Every muscle in his body ached. He rubbed his legs and thought of the past few weeks of cavalry training which was everything that he most abhorred in the handling of horses. Men were treated little better, for they were broken to Army standards as one with the animals they rode.

The instructor, seeing James ride, set him on a rearing black, which to his disgust had obviously come from a bad home, for it had nothing but fear and hatred of its rider. With every move he made, he could still feel its high withers under him from the hours they were made to ride bareback. He pitied the men unused to riding with their bruised crotches and thighs, and calloused hands from the stiff hogged manes beneath the ropes of the bit-less bridles with which they were made to ride. For a large proportion of the day the ruthless training progressed in the riding school in Colwick Park, until the recruits could be called cavalrymen, worthy of the South Notts. Hussars. Although the Hussars advertised for riders, not all made the grade and were transferred unceremoniously to an infantry unit.

James stretched out on his bunk, the rough brown blanket affording some degree of comfort, though not, he thought, to be compared with Ma's soft handmade cotton patchwork quilt on his bed at home. Home. James had endeavoured to keep his mind from what had gone, yet his old way of life persistently infiltrated his thoughts no matter what he was doing, identifying in some way with the path he had chosen. In every face he saw, he looked for Ma and Pa, in every horse, he looked for an O'Malley, yet he would not allow his innermost mind to seek the face of Elizabeth, for nothing he knew, could take away her words which had now become so significant to him: *I would do anything, anything in the world to keep this place.* How could she? He would have taken care of her, worked his fingers to the bone if necessary. If she had ended up penniless it would have made her even more dear to him, were that possible. His gaze was fixed on the wooden beams and boards of the roof above him, had he not been feeling low, he would have stuck to his self-imposed discipline and thrust such thoughts away.

As though taking advantage of his lapse, the memory of Robert Oakley came to his mind. He tried to dispel the image but not before he saw again the man's expression when he had thrown the medallion of St. James at him and spoken those fateful words... They had laughed at him, Oakley and Elizabeth. He cringed at the words he had spoken when he had given her the medallion, 'While ever you wear it, I shall believe that you love me.' Then her reply, 'I'll love you until I die... I vow to Saint James before God that I'll never take it off.' O God... James turned onto his side, his face burning with humiliation.

He deliberately permitted a loud groaning which had been going on for some time to interrupt his thoughts. On the bunk to his right, Fred Preston, a nineteen-year-old farm worker from Lambley, was clutching his groin. James turned to Fred as he spoke. 'How do you feel Jim?' and without waiting for, or expecting a reply, went on. 'Me, I'm ruined for bloody life.'

There was general laughter from around the billet at his words, James smiled wryly.

'See that poor bugger,' Fred nodded his head in the direction of Harry Brown, James' neighbour to his left, who was snoring softly,

'He's had a rough time of it. Can't think what he's doing in this out-fit, his age an' all.' He lit a cigarette and lay back balancing one leg across a raised knee. 'Reckons he was reared on a farm but now he's married with kids he works in a factory.' He lowered his voice. 'Says his wife chafed him to work there, better money and a bonus each year.' He resumed his normal loud tone. 'I'd sooner work outside than be in a factory. Well, if it wasn't been for this bloody war I mean.' He added grinning, drawing on the cigarette he had just lit.

Thinking of the nights he had fallen asleep hearing Fred's voice and the mornings he had woken to it, James closed his mind to the interminable chatter and became aware of other background sounds with which he had become familiar. Groups of men talking around the stove and the occasional burst of laughter, the shake of a dice, the low mumble from card players, a whinny from the stables outside. His thoughts turned to the friend he had made, Toby Mallet, from Hucknall, also under age, who had taken many falls and got up laugh-ing but not so from the last one which had broken his clavicle. Here and there men were writing letters to their loved ones, he had written a few times to put Ma and Pa's minds at rest.

Ma's first letter to him had contained a sentence which had pierced him, something he knew she would never have done inten-tionally. He felt under his mattress and drew out the letter, knowing as he did so that he hardly needed to re-read it, for the words were fixed in his mind. Ma had written, 'Dear James, Pa and I hope you are alright, we wish you hadn't joined up so impulsively, you're too young, do they know that? We miss you so much. You are always in our thoughts and prayers. Please God they don't send you abroad. It's so strange here without you. Everything has changed James. Robert Oakley has agreed to let the place back on rent for now, I would imagine that the two of them talked about it when Elizabeth was poorly and staying at the hall. Mr. Neeson, her solicitor, has insisted on a proper rental agreement, he sees to everything, including the wages. Elizabeth doesn't seem to have any interest at all. We still can't believe what happened, poor John, whatever possessed him?

Dermot got the horses away to Ireland before he left. The yearlings and two-year-olds will stay up in Derbyshire. There are only the trap ponies and remaining farm horses left here which Pa needs for the increased arable. Pa's determined to carry out John's plans. There's a pair of younger farm horses in Derbyshire, which Bob tells us he's breaking in for us. Pa says he'll be glad of them. We shall all have to try and do our best.' Ma had gone on to chastise him for joining up and had pleaded with him to take care of himself, receive the Sacraments regularly and come home safely to them.

James put the letter away. 'The two of them... whilst she was staying at the hall...' It was obvious that Robert Oakley had taken what he considered to be his, which appeared to include Elizabeth, confirming what the man had so cruelly inferred. He had received a strange stilted letter from Elizabeth around the same time, all he could see in it was the influence of Robert Oakley. He had felt patronised and had destroyed it.

The next day, following Reveille at 5am and the horses watered, the long awaited tackle was issued. Stiff new army issue, fit to gall a horse James thought, as along with the others, he oiled, soaped and polished, making little impression on the new leather. Once saddled up, the men sank into the comparative comfort such saddles afforded, albeit without stirrups and found to their amazement that in the main part, they were cavalrymen. This, they considered was the best of the past few weeks, at least they could relax a little, maybe get some time off and see what Nottingham had to offer.

James' first few hours of freedom were spent in the company of Toby Mallet, arm raised in plaster of paris, Fred Preston and Fred's friend, Joe Fletcher, eighteen, from the same village, and Ron Shelton, a nineteen-year-old from Nuthall. They had only managed to get an eight hour pass, so after the horses had been set fair early in the afternoon they had walked to Colwick station and caught the train to Nottingham, the money they had saved during the past few weeks jingling in the pockets of their breeches.

Although James had not been to Nottingham very often, he knew the layout roughly and was able to lead his friends from the railway station to the market place. His first impression was the amount of people in uniform, Army being the most prevalent. Amongst them were nurses and injured servicemen in their distinctive blue suits, white shirts and red ties, which at least, thought James, saved the poor devils from a white feather to add insult to injury. It occurred to him that may well have been the origin of the saying. The town bustled, the numbers of horses surprised him especially after the commandeering of many of the O'Malley's. One law for one... he thought bitterly. The clock on the town hall was striking four as they filed into J. Lyons cafe on Long Row.

'Real food lads,' Fred said tucking into bacon, eggs, sausage and apple pie onto his tray, as did the others, whilst joking and laughing, their spirits high, to the amusement of other diners, a mixed selection of armed forces and elderly civilians. Their immediate needs satisfied they walked out into the market place where gas street lamps had now been lit, illuminating patriotic displays in shop windows, the Union flag and those of the allies much in evidence.

They crossed the market place where the Bell Inn beckoned, a great bell sunk into the wall over the door and made their way into the flagstone passage of one of the oldest pubs in the town, side-stepping to avoid a huge man who was hoisting a barrel of porter. The bar ran the length of the tap room and behind the bar an attractive woman in a high necked lace blouse smiled enquiringly at them as she took hold of one of the pumps, anticipating their order. Joe nodded. 'Five pints of the best, please love.'

There were any amount of pubs around the market and the group called in several before deciding to split up until their walk back to the station later. James, unused to much alcohol felt somewhat disorientated and laughed with Toby about his choice of partner. 'If I fall first you'll never get me up with your crook arm and if you do you'll cut a rare figure laying on your back with that bloody pot sticking up in the air.'

They were still laughing when they passed two girls, James didn't see them at first until Toby nudged him with his good arm and he heard a low giggle from behind.

'See them James, not half bad,' Toby whispered in his ear.

'I didn't notice them.' James didn't look around.

'In that case, I like the other one, not yours.'

James laughed. 'What's wrong with her?'

'Looks stuck up if you ask me.'

Their pace was slowing down and Toby forced a turn on James so that they wandered back past the two girls.

One of them gave the same low giggle. 'What have you been doing then soldier? I've never seen anybody with their arm up there.'

Toby homed in. 'It would take more than a minute to tell you love, how long have you got?'

The girls both laughed at that, the bolder one who had spoken first moved along on the slatted bench upon which they were sitting. 'Here, rest yourself, it must be wearying carrying your arm about like that.'

'I've known better times.'

James stood near the bench amused by the banter.

'Come and sit down Jim, rest your legs.' Toby pulled at his tunic. 'Here, shove up,' he told the girls. 'Make room at the other end for my friend. Ladies, this is Jim Gretton, the finest rider I've had the pleasure to meet.'

'Oh, you broke your arm riding?' The quieter girl spoke for the first time, looking across her friend to Toby whilst at the same time blushing as James sat down beside her.

'If he's Jim, who're you then?' the other girl asked.

'Toby Mallet at your service.'

The girl giggled again, 'I'm Edie and my friend here's Kathy.'

James and Toby nodded in unison. Toby turned to Edie and began a conversation. For a few minutes James sat in silence by Kathy, he smiled inwardly as he realised for the first time in his life what it meant to be hot under the collar. The rough khaki serge of the closed collar of his tunic seemed to stifle him, only by rigid self control did he stop himself from putting a finger around it and admitting some air. He felt the presence of the girl acutely and feeling it was up to him to make some kind of overture, opened his mouth to speak. The girl obviously had the same idea for they both spoke at once and began to laugh.

'After you,' she said lowering her eyes

'No, please, after you,' James said.

'I was going to say that you seem very young to be a soldier.'

'I'm eighteen,' James lied. 'You have to be.'

'A lot are saying that, but it's not always true.'

James let it go. 'Do you live in Nottingham?'

'Yes, at the top of Alfreton Road, well, one of the streets off there, Raleigh Street, it's not far, do you know it?'

'Is it near the arboretum?'

'Fairly near. Do you know the arboretum then?'

'Not really, it's just that someone I went to Sunday school with lives near to it. Florence Smith, do you know her?'

'No, sorry. Do you keep in touch?'

'Sort of. Someone else who went does, they write to each other and exchange visits and so I've seen her now and then, kept in touch that way.' Through Elizabeth, he thought in exasperation, how and why had he managed to bring the past into it. He fell silent and stared down at the ground, cursing himself.

'Are you alright?' Kathy asked, tilting her head towards him.

He looked up at her and smiled. 'Yes, of course.'

In the gaslight she looked pale, her eyes luminous, a slip of light brown hair escaping from her bonnet gave her an air of vulnerability and he wanted to reach out and tuck it back. Instead, he listened to her voice which was low and soft and had none of her friend's brittleness.

'No, I don't usually do this sort of thing,' she was saying. 'You see Edie is always asking me to come out, meet some of the soldiers, she says it's only right that we should try and cheer up the boys going to war,' she blushed again. 'That's what Edie says anyway.'

'I'm sure she's right,' James agreed, his eyes still on her face. 'You've certainly cheered me up.'

The bench gave a little as Edie and Toby stood up. James looked at Toby questioningly. Toby winked, 'Tell you what Jim, I'll meet you with the others later, me and Edie's going for a walk, she's going to show me the town.'

The girl beside James stood up abruptly, 'I must be going now.'

He could see that she was ill at ease being alone with him, he didn't want her to leave, the thought of it made him feel desolate. He stood by her and caught her hand. 'Don't go Kathy, stay, talk to me, please.' She hesitated. 'I'll not harm you.'

Slowly, she sat down again, James beside her. He encouraged her to talk about herself, gradually feeling her relax. She told him of her work in a factory manufacturing Nottingham lace and of her mother and small brothers and sisters, of their struggle since her father had joined up and of the hours she helped her mother do lace work at home, drawing threads and preparing the lace to be carded.

'We're always covered in bits of cotton,' she said laughing. 'I'll bet I could find some on me now, it's messy work.'

'You look perfect to me,' he said sincerely. 'I can't see any bits on you.'

She blushed and looked down at her neat buttoned boots, only raising her eyes after he began to tell her a little about his training so far in the Hussars, making light of it, though nothing of his former life. For a while they fell silent and she looked up at the town hall clock. 'I really must go now Jim.'

'I'll walk with you if you'd like me to,' James offered and they stood awkwardly not touching, then walked side by side, Kathy taking him in the direction of her home. They left the market place via Chapel Bar and made their way up Derby Road, passing the great

Cathedral of St. Barnabas and on up the hill to where the road divided, an area of land known as Canning Circus.

'Something smells good,' James commented stopping for a moment.

'Wilson's chip stall,' she told him eagerly. 'They're the best chips in town, some say for miles around.'

They made their way through a throng of people who were huddled around a large white canvas awning which hung high over coke fires. Chips were frying in bubbling fat in great tinned copper pans.

'Watch Charlie Wilson and you'll soon see why the chips are so good.' James watched as the chips were lifted in a wire basket out of the fat, shaken well and the basket placed on a wire rack by the side of the fire.

'That's called blanching,' she explained. 'Then they go back into the hot fat.' She spoke up. 'Fried in pure lard, aren't they Mr. Wilson?'

The man glanced in their direction and recognised her. 'So they are Kathy, the same as my Ma's chips on her stall down Parliament Street.'

Kathy nodded proudly to James, 'You see.'

James smiled at her. 'How many shall we have then?'

Kathy blushed. 'Oh I didn't mean...'

'But we must sample the best chips in Nottingham and how about some for the little 'uns?'

'They'd like that, if that's alright I mean.'

'Course it is.'

A handsome woman with striking green eyes took James' order and filled several paper boats with crisp golden chips.

'Could you leave two open and wrap the rest please Mrs. Wilson? We're taking some home.'

She did as Kathy asked, accepting the money from James as she looked him over and nodded her approval to Kathy. The girl blushed and busied herself with the paper parcel and her own boat of chips. They ate in silence, their faces red and glowing from the heat of the fires.

James looked about him, how different he thought, Canning Circus looked by night, the darkness shutting out the almshouses, livery stables and horse trough. He recalled his rare trips into Nottingham in the past when Pa and he would bring a pony and trap, leaving the pony at the livery stables whilst they did their business in the town. It was about the only part of Nottingham he really knew well. It seemed strange to be standing there now, isolated in a little world of warmth and comfort. He found the chips were all Kathy had promised and he held one up to her and nodded grinning before he slowly ate it with great relish. She laughed and he kept his eyes on her, studying her in the firelight and he saw that she was neatly dressed, slim and small boned. She became aware of his gaze and dropped her eyes and he recognised her shyness which Toby had mistaken for stand-offishness. He decided that she was quite unaware of her attraction, of her sheer femininity, which was balm to him after the harshness of the past few weeks and the desperate hurt which had been inflicted upon him prior to that.

Their paper boats emptied, he offered his arm as he walked her home and after a while she slipped her arm through his, hesitantly. They turned into a street of Victorian terraced houses and she stopped in front of one of them. The feeling of desolation stole over him again.

'Will you meet me next week if I can get leave, the same time and place as we met tonight?' he rushed his words, his eyes not leaving her face. 'Only if you want to,' he added hastily.

She nodded, looking up at him. 'Yes.' she said quietly, beginning to climb the steps to the front door where she stopped and turned. 'Thank you for a nice evening Jim.' Then she was gone and he was alone in the street.

James and Kathy were destined not to meet again.

❧ ❧ ❧

During December, the recruits joined the Regiment in Norfolk. An enemy landing on the east coast was expected a few days before

Christmas. The task of the South Notts. Hussars along with other Yeomanry and Territorial units was 'to stand guard over the homes and fields of England.'

On the afternoon of 23rd December, all leave was stopped and the Regiment stood under arms for seven hours. James' Squadron, 'B', based at Salterhouse had to wade through water up to their knees to get to their posts, it was bitterly cold and at intervals, the men walked their chilled horses around for exercise.

On Christmas Eve the Regiment were at the ready for instant parade. In the early hours of Christmas morning another assembly was called and when dawn broke on the ranks of the South Notts. they were surrounded by a hard white frost. Again, the Regiment stood ready for seven hours. The enemy did not invade.

XIV

JANUARY, 1915

The windows of the train were wet with condensation. Elizabeth wiped the one beside her with her glove and stared out, watching the fields rush by as Nottinghamshire gave way to Derbyshire. The sky was heavy with snow and she hoped to get her business done with Bob Sherwin at Gatthorpe and return before the weather broke. She was accompanied by Aunt Martha, who had been a pillar of strength and with whom she was now living in Lincoln for the duration of the war.

The torment with which Elizabeth lived was foremost in her mind and for the millionth time she asked herself why James had left. She had been over and over the last time they had been together when he had told her of his plans. Going away definitely did not feature in them. *Why, why, why?* She bit her lip. *He couldn't have loved me.* The rhythm of the wheels rolling over the tracks mocked her, *He couldn't have done, he couldn't have done.* A heavy tear rolled down her cheek and she kept her face averted, her gaze fixed on the window as she stared out, unseeing, bewilderment causing to her feel hollow inside.

After a while she made herself think over the past few months. Following discussions with Mr. Neeson, Tom, Dermot and her aunt, it had been agreed to apply to rent the stud farm back from Robert Oakley. This option Elizabeth felt, seemed to be the best thing they could do under the circumstances and also, she admitted to herself, it helped defer the loss. She was also aware that renting would enable Tom to carry out John's plans, which Tom was confident would show good returns. Through his solicitor and agent, Robert Oakley had agreed and although they all felt that the tenancy was somewhat tenuous and only granted because of the war, a five year tenancy agreement had been finally settled upon. Tom and Annie would be secure at least for five years and Mrs. Bailey could stay on at the house, as caretaker.

Through the reflection in the window, she saw her aunt glance at her as she put down the *Punch* magazine she was reading and remove her spectacles. 'You are quiet Elizabeth, are you alright my dear?'

Elizabeth nodded and turned from the window. She knew that her eyes were still bright with tears for James. 'Yes aunt, I'm alright. My mind seems to be in turmoil with recent events and I was miles away, thinking my way through them.'

'That's a good thing to do, file them as it were, in one's mind. I'm sure we've all made the right decisions given the circumstances, but truly Elizabeth, my priority now, is to see you restored to your usual health and vitality.'

Elizabeth reached out her hand and held that of her aunt for a moment as she looked into her aunt's eyes. 'I'll try not to fail you then,' she said with the suggestion of a smile. Once her aunt was re-immersed in her reading, Elizabeth resumed her thoughts, with purpose now as she appreciated her aunt's practicality regarding them.

She thought with gratitude of her Irish relatives and of Dermot staying until the last of the three-year-olds and brood mares were safely in Ireland. Some were to be sold, the rest staying at the Sullivan Bloodstock Agency. The brood mares either visiting selected stallions or awaiting foaling and the service of her new stallion. Tom and the Sullivans' had made an intensive search for a top class entire and had assured her that she would be impressed by their choice. Scamall, an eight-year-old grey stallion of excellent breeding, temperament and confirmation, with a good fertility record. He was by Solgar, the well reputed English thoroughbred stallion standing at the Curragh and out of a powerful Irish Draft mare. She herself had not yet seen Scamall and was to travel to Ireland with Tom on his next visit.

She was looking forward to the prospect of some horse business with Tom, for although moved by his continuing commitment to her father's plans with the increased arable venture, and whilst giving him her full support, she could raise no enthusiasm for the project.

Bob Sherwin met them at Chesterfield with a pony and trap and Elizabeth re-introduced her aunt to him, for they had already met at the recent funerals.

'Best put these rugs over your knees, Miss Elizabeth, ma'am,' he nodded to Elizabeth and Martha in turn as he passed wool rugs to them. 'It's perishing cold up here,' he said taking the reins and driving out of the station yard.

'How are the youngsters Bob?'

'Right as rain. Can't beat Derbyshire grazing.'

Elizabeth thought with nostalgia of the same words her father had spoken so often. She pulled a rug around her and shivered.

'Aye, it's going to come,' Bob said succinctly, looking up at the leaden sky. 'I was hoping Tom would be with you, it's a fair way for you ladies on your own.'

'They're busy threshing Bob, the machine was already booked and he's got the worry of the weather breaking up. He's very committed to this project of Papa's. The grain we would have used for our own horses, with the exception of the feed we send up here, is to be sold to the War Office and he plans to increase the output next year. There's only Tom, the two older men and a few of the lads left now.' She didn't voice Tom's concerns regarding them making the trip without him.

They drove through the village and began the climb to Upper Gatthorpe, Bob slowing the pony to a walk, and as they rounded a bend the holding came into view. O'Malley land stretched around the Jacobean farmhouse, cottage and outbuildings, which sat as solid as the Derbyshire stone from which they were built. Elizabeth's great-grandfather had been prudent in adding large stone and wooden sheds which afforded the horses shelter from the relentless wind from the high peaks.

Bob's wife, Amy, greeted them, making a great fuss of Elizabeth and bustling them into the parlour where a roaring log fire blazed.

'I know you'll want to get out to the stock Miss Elizabeth,' she plumped a cushion up behind Elizabeth's back urging her to be comfortable, 'but I've made a batch of nice meat pasties and some leek soup and I would feel happier to see you eat something before you do. Warm you up after your journey.' She looked to Martha for support, who nodded her agreement.

A short time later Elizabeth went out with Bob to see the yearlings and two-year-olds.

'They look a picture,' Elizabeth complimented him as she walked slowly through the sheds, consulting the file she had brought with her. 'They've grown on well.' She stroked the muzzle of an enquiring yearling, 'Dimity's foal, unless I'm mistaken?'

Bob smiled. 'You're right, she's a beauty isn't she? By Bladhaire, he's thrown some good 'uns. It's a damn shame you've lost Ri Rua, Tom tells me he was going from strength to strength.'

'He was. He had developed into a magnificent animal. He had it all, temperament, confirmation and had to be the best horse I've ever ridden.'

'Well, you've certainly ridden some, I should think as far back as you can remember.'

Elizabeth nodded, 'I don't remember learning to ride and the same with James. He said that riding Rua was like riding the west wind.' She looked at him. 'It was all so terrible Bob, losing any of them, but I don't think I shall ever get over losing Rua.' Or James, she thought, but made an effort at normality for Bob's sake.

'I can understand that,' he said shaking his head sadly and as if reading her thoughts, added, 'I couldn't get over it when I heard about James joining up. What was he, sixteen?' Elizabeth nodded.

'So young, it must have broken Tom and Annie's hearts. It nearly did ours when our eldest went, but at least he was nineteen. Not that age makes any difference to how you miss them.' He adjusted a headstall on one of the youngsters and fondled its ears.

'No,' Elizabeth said quietly and making an effort to turn the conversation, asked him. 'How are you going to manage Bob? Annie tells me that two of the lads have enlisted as well as your son.'

'I've done what Tom advised and managed to get a couple of older men in to help, one's had experience in racing stables and the other was a local hunt servant, so along with our younger son, I should manage. The work load's always that much lighter every year when the three-year-olds go down to you at the stud. I know they haven't this year, they've gone to Ireland instead. That's left us with forty-two young 'uns here, after John sold some of the geldings. I can always get some retired help in if we're pushed.'

As they progressed around the young stock, Bob marvelled at Elizabeth's incredible memory of their breeding. He had been aware of this since she was a child when she accompanied her father on his frequent visits to the holding. He sighed, those were the days, a family devoted to their horses and by God they'd bred some clouters, 'chasers, point to pointers, hunters, all highly coveted and how many studs had started out with O'Malley foundation stock? Countless. He watched Elizabeth's face as she passed from one to the other, consulting the files for which she had no need. Pure absorption, he thought, she's totally lost to the world and for a while, to the tragedies which had been inflicted upon her.

'You do well Bob, you always have. They're a big responsibility for you,' she said eventually, putting her hand on his arm.

'Don't you worry about anything Miss Elizabeth, these horses up here and them you're keeping over in Ireland will pull you through after the war, you'll see. It would have been madness to leave them all in this country with the possibility of commandeering every so often, not to mention deliberately letting brood mares go barren. It's been a miracle we've been able to ship them off without somebody taking it on themselves to interfere, perhaps whoever it was who tipped them off in the first place.'

Elizabeth looked at him, but he gave no indication as to whom he might have been referring. She no longer doubted James' suspicion.

'I do so appreciate everything you are all doing for me.'

He shuffled his feet in embarrassment as she continued, 'Tom's there for you and we'll all keep in touch with each other every few weeks, if you need me in between you've only to write. Mr. Neeson will see to wages, expenses and anything you may require, so he'll be in regular contact.' Elizabeth put her hand out to him and he grasped it firmly.

XV

Robert made a half hearted attempt to pull off his boots, they were wet to a point of being soggy and he saw to his annoyance that his hands were covered in mud.

'Smith,' he called irritably, 'where in hell's name are you?'

A cheery whistle preceded the appearance of a dapper, lively individual.

'Yes captain,' he spoke in the unmistakable accent of the East End.

Robert held out his legs in disdain. 'For God's sake rid me of these foul boots, and,' he added, glowering at the man, 'be careful.'

Quietly whistling a couple more impudent bars, Smith gave an almighty pull at the left boot. Robert cursed him soundly, rolling his eyes to the ceiling. He gazed idly around the room, which was quite the largest in the small hotel in which they were billeted. It boasted a half tester bed and basic bathing facilities behind an ornate Louis fifteenth style screen. He supposed it could be worse, the village was some four miles behind the lines. Not, he felt, that he was having an easy time with his responsibility for supplies, for his greatest concern, next to self preservation, was that there was not nearly enough of them.

He remembered, not so long ago, when the allies had to leave off retaliating to enemy fire, because there hadn't been enough ammunition. God Almighty, it had been an absolute disgrace. He knew that munitions were now priority at home, yet still hand to mouth on the battlefield. The enemy had been arming for years, it was bloody outrageous. He sighed with relief as his right boot slid off, reminding Smith to get them onto boot trees immediately. Smith gave him a resentful glance as he fitted in the trees which bore the name of a well known Melton Mowbray bootmaker.

'Is there any hot water?'

'I've got what I could captain, it's in the bath ready for you.'

A few seconds later, Robert's head appeared around the screen. 'Bloody hell man, how long ago did you get the water? Come in here at once.' Smith sauntered over to the screen, Robert was standing with a towel around his waist eyeing two or three inches of tepid water in a hip bath with disdain.

Smith was aggrieved. 'Captain, I don't think you realise what a job I've had to get you a bath at all, they're very reluctant to part with any hot water in the kitchen.'

'Are they indeed,' Robert stirred the water with his toe. 'You can do something about that for tomorrow evening.' Smith opened his mouth to retaliate, but closed it as Robert waved him away.

Once seated in the bath, making do with its abysmal contents, Robert had to admit to himself that despite Smith's cunning and idleness, on the whole he was an excellent scrounger. Anything that could be made into a palatable meal found its way onto Robert's table each evening and he had learned it was wiser not to over pursue the origin. Smith, he knew, had seen to it that his superior was respected in the small French village, glibly creating the impression that only one such as his captain could fortify the village against the enemy. It was therefore hardly surprising that the few cottagers who had not fled from the advancing Germans rallied patriotically to the interests and stomach of the brave English Captain.

Had Robert but realised, he and his soldier servant were very much alike, not maybe in appearance, one elegant and educated, the other a sly survivor from the slums of dockland, for each possessed the priority of self. Smith had learned through the craft of rough living, Robert by the easy acceptance of years of faithful ministrations by old and trusted servants.

Dinner that night consisted mainly of boiled fowl, old and stringy maybe, but certainly more acceptable than the eternal bully beef hashed up in the trenches and eaten in the face of enemy fire. Robert drained the bottle of local wine into his glass and drank it, spluttering over the heavy sediment and spitting most of it onto the bones of the fowl. He wiped his mouth on the back of his hand cursing Smith for his lack of finesse in not decanting it in some way and also not providing him with a napkin. What would he not give for some decent cheese followed by a good brandy. It was bloody ludicrous to be here in France with none of the basics. Robert sat back in his chair pondering the inevitable question of how to fill in the long evening ahead. He dismissed the idea of writing home, news of the war was so heavily censored that it left little to write about.

There was no longer any need to issue further instructions to his solicitor and agent, as the transfer of John O'Malley Sullivan's house and land had been successfully completed some time ago. He suppressed a smirk as he thought of the O'Malley family's pathetic attempts to thwart him, why, even their own solicitor, that old fool Neeson had to concede that his ownership of the O'Malley Sullivan holding at Oakley was quite legitimate and as for the absurd behaviour of his father, he deserved all he had got. Robert laughed aloud as he recalled the fateful card game; he'd had that stupid drunken fool in the palm of his hand.

By God, he'd sorted out Miss Elizabeth all right, he was determined to possess her and had been since the night of the ball when she had been in the company of that dolt, Brown. He congratulated himself, things were working out better than he could have anticipated, she'd be in no doubt now who had the whip hand. He felt almost benevolent that he had permitted her to rent the place, although he had to admit, that he had been surprised by the request. Placing herself under an obligation to him would give him the best of both worlds, Elizabeth living in her old home, whilst he was the owner of it. Robert laughed again. A five year tenancy was not the end of the world and he would no doubt have had his use of her by then leaving him the pleasure of showing her, along with the remaining O'Malley retainers where to get off and the first to go would be the ex-stud groom and his bastard, who'd had the temerity to hang around Elizabeth.

'Captain,' Smith's voice followed a tap on the door, interrupting his musings.

'Clear off damn you, I was half asleep.'

Sighing ill-humouredly, Robert trained his thoughts back to his treatment of Elizabeth on the day of his father's stroke. Soon he was experiencing again the euphoria he had felt from the heavy blow he had inflicted on the side of her face, seeing again the whiteness of her neck and breast as he tore her blouse from her shoulder. For a while he indulged himself in anticipation of his plans for her. Marry Victoria, he thought, no point whatsoever in marrying Elizabeth O'Malley Sullivan, not only was she a papist but he already had the bulk of her inheritance and now she'd be no more than a grateful puppet to his whims. He sank deeper into his reverie, hearing again her gasp, seeing the pain in her eyes as he ripped that ridiculous medal from her neck. It had been all he could do to leave her and ride off for the doctor, when every instinct had been to throw her onto her back and force himself upon her. Beads of sweat broke out on his forehead at the prospect, whilst he had to make do recalling the exquisite pleasure he had obtained from his treatment of her that day. Yes, he reaffirmed, stroking his body sensuously, marry that simpering creature Victoria with her massive inheritance but be cautious of his treatment of her in bed in the knowledge of a willing rape who lived close by, no doubt anxious to submit to his every whim in order to take whatever crumbs he offered. His body now aroused, would not lie dormant. The thought of playing a hand or two of cards with Smith held no appeal for him at all.

There was another knock at the door, this time more urgent. 'Captain, the landlord's invited you down to the bar.' There was a silence, followed by Smith's voice taking on a wheedling tone. 'He sent me 'specially to ask you to join him.'

Bored and indifferent, Robert drifted down the stairs, at least he might be able to prise from the landlord several glasses of the excellent wine he knew to have been hidden away when his regiment had first entered the village. To his surprise the landlord was in conversation with two girls, one of whom lowered her eyes, blushing in awe at Robert's presence, the other held her head up brazenly and looked at him appraisingly. He relaxed. After many months he was again in the position he enjoyed at home, venerated by the local inhabitants. He smiled, his most charming smile. *'Bonsoir, Mesdemoiselles. Comment allez-vous?'*

They giggled together, the elder and more confident, shook her frizzy flaxen hair over her shoulder and gave him a dazzling smile. *'Bonsoir, M'suir le Capitan.'*

Robert recognised the type as universal. She thrust her large breasts close to him just nudging his arm and held his gaze for a while, her eyes wide and full of promise. Robert squared his shoulders whilst the landlord, smiling to himself, produced a vessel containing the much coveted wine and four glasses.

The evening proved a pleasant one and when Smith had occasion to pass through the room, slyly winking at the younger girl, Robert actually prided himself on the newly acquired discretion of the man. Shortly afterwards the girl excused herself and left via the same door through which Smith had significantly departed. Tactfully the landlord suddenly found some pressing duties to occupy him elsewhere and Robert had no difficulty in persuading the now befuddled girl to accompany him to his room, taking what was left of the wine with them.

After she had departed, Robert lay on his back smoking, not displeased with the agreeable turn the evening had taken. He smiled as he stubbed the half smoked cigarette into the ashtray. She'd taken a fair bit of roughing up prior to his gratification, he recalled with satisfaction. Amazing what these stupid bitches would put up with if he threw enough francs at them, though, in the dimness of the room, he had not perpetrated his sadism upon her, but upon a dark haired girl many miles away.

Out in the barn, Smith was also smiling. His ruse had worked very well. Admittedly, it had cost him some of the captain's cigarettes, but didn't he always endeavour to obtain good provision for any of the captain's possessions? The girl spread-eagled on Captain Oakley's groundsheet giggled as Smith devoted his attention to her. He was not articulate in the girl's language, but was well frequented with a more universal one. He could never have had the entire evening with Cherie, had they not contrived to distract the captain with Jeanne.

XVI

APRIL TO NOVEMBER, 1915

James tied up his horse in the stall allocated to him below decks of the *S.S. Saturnia,* docked at Avonmouth. The hold was bustling with men performing the same duties amid an air of expectancy. Orders that the South Notts. Hussars along with the Derbyshire, Worcestershire and Warwickshire Yeomanry Regiments and a squadron of the Royal Gloucestershire Yeomanry, were to embark for Egypt, sailing the following day, 8th April, had raised morale, certainly amongst the Hussars, James thought, as he stroked a body brush over the bay gelding. The inactivity during the past months in Norfolk was over, along with the petty inspections and monotonous hours of coastal vigilance. The inactivity on board, James considered, was bound to be quite different, for when the horses were seen to and inspection over, there would surely be time to mingle with comrades old and new and enjoy a certain amount of freedom on the voyage.

This proved to be so, and four days out, he was joined at the rails by Toby Mallet whose face James noted was maintaining the pale shade of green to which it had turned, after only two hours at sea.

'Feeling better?' he asked

'Terrible, If I'd known about this lot I'd have never enlisted. I wouldn't have believed I could be so sick, even when there was nothing left in my stomach, I couldn't stopped retching. I hate the sea, it'll be the death of me.'

'Don't say that Tobe, you'll get over it, you are doing already.'

Toby stood with his back to the rails and threaded his arms through them. 'God Jim you're so lucky not to be amongst the lot in the sick bay, the place stinks.'

'Think of the horses, some of those poor sods are sea sick. Horses can't physically vomit, so imagine what they're suffering.'

'God help them, I've noticed some are looking badly. Thanks for doing my horse Jim, I just don't know how I would have coped if you hadn't carried me about the last few days.'

'Do you want to come below and see your horse?' James asked him.

'Not if you say he's alright, I'm better huddling in a corner keeping my eyes shut.' He closed them meaningly as he went on, 'What do you think we're going into then?'

'It's got to be Gallipoli.'

'The Turks are ruthless aren't they?'

'So they say,' James kept his eyes on the horizon.

'Does it bother you?'

James shrugged knowing that a few months ago it would have done, but not so much now. He looked into the pale youthful face of Toby his eyes closed against the swell and realised that any foreboding he felt was more for him.

᪥ ᪥ ᪥

As dawn broke on the 24th April the vessel docked at Alexandria and the Yeomanry Regiments disembarked forthwith and proceeded to the Abbassia Main Barracks, Cairo, where they were quartered until 20th July when they were moved to Kasr-el-Nil.

James with a small group of other Hussars, lay back on a dune smoking. The sun had gone down and they were now used to the considerable drop in temperature with the swift descent of night.

'At least the bloody flies are paralysed with cold,' Ron Shelton said.

'They're not the only ones,' Harry Brown held his cigarette in his mouth whilst he rubbed his hands vigorously together. 'I was thinking it would be romantic to have my wife out here, lying looking up at the stars together, but she wouldn't like it, especially the perishing cold nights. I've always had to see she'd got a good fire and plenty of coal in. Also nice warm clothes, she likes clothes, she's very smart is Vera,' he added self consciously.

Fred Preston nudged Joe Fletcher in the ribs as he stifled a laugh and whispered in Joe's ear. 'Poor Harry, I reckon he must have carried that woman about, he's always on about her.'

'I know, talks of nothing much else, it's enough to put you off marriage for life.'

Harry continued, oblivious to their quiet exchange of words. 'The pattern of stars is so different out here to England, I can't recognise any of them.'

'That's true, it makes you realise how far we are from home.' James said, closing his eyes, fighting off the memories which flooded into his mind. He and Elizabeth lying out in the hot summer nights, watching the stars come out over Oakley, identifying the Sickle and Milky Way. He could feel her presence and hear her voice. He still ached for her. For Elizabeth as she was then, he told himself angrily, not the girl who had spurned him so ruthlessly through a man she knew he detested. He stood up abruptly, grinding the stub of his cigarette into the sand. 'Going to check the horses before I turn in.'

'They're alright Jim, settle down, get a break while you can.' Ron Shelton rolled over onto his stomach, sliding down the dune. 'Oh bloody hell, sand's pouring into my pants, another night of grit where it most hurts.'

The others in the group laughed, but James had already left.

The following day rumours began to spread that the Mounted Division was to be sent as infantry to Gallipoli and by the 8th August orders to this effect were received, but cancelled a few hours later. On the 11th August orders came suddenly for the Yeomanry to proceed to the Dardanelles, dismounted. Two composite squadrons were to be formed, each to consist of some 160 non-commissioned officers and men and six officers, while four officers and 100 other ranks were to be left with the horses in Egypt.

James' Squadron 'B' along with 'D' Squadron were fitted out with infantry equipment two days before leaving for Alexandria, their destination being Suvla Bay.

✂ ✂ ✂

James could hardly breathe, 360 South Notts. Hussars had been packed like herrings on a Clyde steamboat at Mudros at nightfall. There was barely room to stand, but stand they had to, all night, seeing up the coast of the peninsula flashes from guns and rifles, for most of them their first sight of enemy fire. The disembarkation was just before dawn by picket boats and the regiment marched about a mile up the beach before digging in. The shelling they had seen from sea became more intense with daybreak, causing the first of their casualties. No sooner had they settled in than they were moved again and once more had to dig themselves in. There had been no sleep the night before on the crowded steamboat and the men were exhausted, pick and shovel work being new to the majority of the troopers.

Along with the other men of his squadron, James lay in the bottom of a trench, listening to the whispers around him. The silence of the night was interrupted at intervals by shell fire.

'Bastards,' Ron Shelton muttered, 'every time I drop off I nearly jump out of my skin.'

'That's why they do it,' Harry Brown muttered.

'Is this the beach where all those troops were killed in April?' Toby's voice came hoarsely from the other side of James.

'That was at Helles and Anzac. One of the officers was saying that we're a few miles north of Anzac.' James tried to reassure him. 'I suppose it will always be known as Anzac Cove from now on, after Australian and New Zealand Amy Corps who attacked the Western Coast. It was known before as Ari Buru.'

'A massacre...' a trooper started to say before James nudged him in the ribs, mindful of Toby.

Surely one of the worst massacres in history, James thought, refraining from further comment, having heard that 84,000 German trained Turks led by German officers under the command of General

Liman von Sanders, had been waiting for the poor bastards. He offered Toby a drink from his flask, feeling sympathy for his friend who had already suffered a broken collar bone and chronic sea sickness and was still listless and not well. He seemed to James to be so much younger than he, for all they had both reached their seventeenth birthday since joining up.

By 20th August the South Notts. had been moved to Lala Baba for the battle of Scimitar Hill the following day, under the command of Major Barber, the main objective to secure Anafarta Heights. As the regiment advanced across open ground on the right of Salt Lake, they saw the leading regiments before them suffer a great deal of casualties and the South Notts. passed over many dead and wounded, another new experience for the majority. To make matters worse, the shrub caught fire, burning many of the wounded to death. The Yeomanry Regiments including the South Notts. Hussars, marched shoulder to shoulder, closing ranks as clusters of them were taken out by shellfire. As darkness fell, the survivors had no choice but to return to the trenches.

James re-tied the filthy bandage on his left upper arm, holding one end of it in his teeth. Shrapnel had taken half an inch of flesh on the outer side in a wound about three inches long. A bandage around his head covered a multitude of smaller shrapnel wounds.

A trooper by his side, left off cleaning his gun. 'Do you want any help with that? Though you'd be better going back to the dressing station.'

'No thanks, I can manage,' James spoke through his teeth.

'You're a lucky bastard,' the trooper observed. 'That piece of shell could have been in your heart. Bloody Turks, they ain't got hearts so you'd wonder how they know where to aim.' He leaned back on the side of the trench and resumed his task.

'I'll never know how any of us survived.'

'Me neither, it was nothing but butchery. They didn't completely get away with it though, them in front who got to the enemy trenches bayoneted as many as they could, one of the few who made it back said they ran down the other side of the hill after the Turks who had escaped. But not many of our lads made it back up the hill afterwards, more's the pity.'

'By God, Jim, we thought neither you nor Toby had made it,' Harry Brown joined in shaking his head.

James put his shirt on and carefully eased his injured arm into the sleeve. The cloth was ripped and bloody, his fingernails were black with dried blood. He had nothing to change into as they had brought only what they could carry on the steamer.

'Joe Fletcher and Fred Preston didn't,' James lowered his head, seeing again the multitude of fallen, amongst them the two comrades who had crumpled like bloody broken dolls by his side. For a moment he had glanced sideways and knew he would remember the expression on Joe's face for the rest of his life, the appaling shock followed by indescribable agony which had caused him to scream aloud as half of the upper part of his body was ripped away. In those seconds Joe had seemed incredulously aware of his ghastly mutilation, the shattered rib cage and shreds of tattered flesh. Fred, reduced to a bloody tangled mess, fell beside him.

Since then James had been in torment because he hadn't been able to do anything for them, not even the basic humanity of stopping, the relentless march across the open plain had continued. He recalled hearing Toby cry out and had elbowed him behind, giving him the scant protection of his right shoulder, yet at the same time that Joe and Fred, had fallen to his left, he had felt the searing heat as a fragment of shrapnel had torn into his arm and fall out from the shell had peppered his head. He had staggered on but hadn't the strength in his left arm to raise his rifle at the top of the hill and in trying, had fallen writhing on the ground as Toby had dropped across him.

Harry's voice broke into his thoughts. 'Yes, by God, we were sure you'd both had it.'

James shuddered, he remembered the thud of a fallen man's rifle butt on the back of his head as more weight descended on him. Then the slow return to consciousness, the awareness of awful suffering around him, the crackle of fire and the appalling stench of roasting flesh. He rubbed the heel of his right hand into his eyes and felt the bile rising again in his throat as it had done the previous night. Amongst the sound of sobbing and gibbering he had recognised the voice of Toby lying across him, shaking uncontrollably and crying for his mother.

He remembered the tremendous effort he had made to crawl out of the hill of bodies, amongst shattered bone, torn flesh and fabric, blood and viscera. His left arm had hurt abominably with the effort but he persevered, clawing himself out. Then dragging Toby from underneath and holding him in his arms and calming him until he could get him to crawl down the hill in the darkness, avoiding the large patches of scrub fires which would have made easy targets of them from above. He looked at Toby now, sitting in water on the floor of the trench, rocking backwards and forwards, trembling at intervals. A couple of the other men followed James' eyes and shook their heads.

'They say that a lot of ours are still on one of the hills, Ron Shelton maybe amongst them. There don't seem many of us left here.'

'Chances are they've had it.'

'The terrible thing is that there's still wounded out there, the medical officer and volunteers did what they could after dark, but none of us can do anything until nightfall again.'

'Aye, crawling from body to body, trying to get some response.'

'It was sheer carnage, they used us for cannon fodder to distract the enemy fire from the big guns on the battleships in the harbour.'

The men fell silent. James tied off his bandage, he knew what they said was true. As they had marched across the open plain towards the enemy's advantage points on top of the hill, he had known it for sure. Behind them thousands watched with field glasses, while bombarding the enemy from the sea. Whatever strategy had been planned, they had been sacrificed as part of it.

The Battle of Scimitar Hill was the last Gallipoli offensive, though it had failed through no fault of the troops. The casualties of the

Yeomanry Division were stated to be 1,200, nearly a quarter of its strength, the total casualties being some 12,000 in killed, wounded and missing.

The conditions in the trenches at Suvla were appaling, as the entire line was under the full observation of the Turks who occupied the higher ground and their guns could fire on any front. The trenches were in an unsanitary condition, in many places down to water at three feet, which was the only drinking water available. There were hundreds of dead bodies around and swarms of flies descended upon the men's diet of bully beef and biscuits. The men began to go down with dysentery and para-typhoid, their faces covered with swarms of flies which they had no energy to brush away. They were still wearing what they had on when they left for Suvla Bay on 20th August. Men died wretched deaths, in the filth of the trenches, in the squalor of the latrines, body piled upon body, their rot sustaining millions more flies to infect the rest. James boiled drops of water in a bully beef tin and struggled to keep Toby and himself from disease, yet despite his valiant attempts, they both succumbed to bouts of dysentery.

On the night of 2nd November, the remnant of James' regiment struggled to the vessel, *Ermine*. The evacuation of Gallipoli was under way. The Allies had suffered 180,000 casualties.

XVII

OAKLEY, 1916

In his usual manner, Saxon banged the gate of the top yard noisily behind him. 'Beth,' he shouted in the general direction of the house, his voice ringing through the empty yard. He strode towards the door as Tom appeared from the back of the stables.

'Morning Saxon, how are you?'

'Fine Mr Sharkey, and yourself?'

'Bearing up, all things considered.' Tom jerked his thumb in the direction of the stables with their closed and bolted doors.

Saxon shook his head ruefully. 'Is Elizabeth around?'

'Should be, she and her aunt have been here for a few days, we've been to see Bob and the stock up in Derbyshire.'

'Yes, she wrote and told me, everything alright up there?'

'Fine, thanks.'

Saxon raised his hand, then leapt up the steps to the house, and banged hard on the knocker.

'Lord in his mercy, whatever can be so urgent?' Aunt Martha held her hand to her chest as the banging on the door continued. Elizabeth ran down the stairs, patting her aunt's arm reassuringly as she passed by to open the front door. Saxon poised for another assault on the knocker grinned at her.

'Oh Saxon, you frightened us to half to death. Come along in. It's lovely to see you.' She took his hand and pulled him into the hall.

'And you Beth, I was pleased as punch to hear you were coming over. Came to see if you would like to come for a stroll with me?' Without waiting for her reply, he urged. 'Go and get something warm on. It's a perfect winter's day, but very cold.'

'I know, I took the dogs for a run first thing. Would you like a cup of tea before we go?'

'We'll have one when we come back shall we?'

Elizabeth sat him in the drawing room whilst she sped off, reappearing seconds later in a thick warm coat with a wide woollen scarf around her head. The village road was completely white and their footsteps disturbed delicate billows of powdery frost. Elizabeth slipped her arm through Saxon's and he drew her to him as he might have done a puppy or small animal, patting her hand. They chatted as they walked, turning without comment into the bridle path, where, although the pale winterly sun was filtering through the bare branches of the beech trees, the faded clumps of grass beneath them were still crusted with frost and in the ruts of the path ice crackled beneath their feet.

'So how's Lincoln really suiting you then Beth?'

'Better than I thought it would. My aunt is such kind, easy company, yet at the same time very intelligent and interesting. Mama always admired Aunt Martha's intellect.'

'Your Mama had an intellect of her own,' Saxon said with feeling.

'She's like Mama in so many ways and she's done so much for me. It's only recently that I've realised how ill I really must have been when she first took me home with her.'

'You'd had enough to make you and then the final straw of having your home stolen from you by that swine... it's beyond comprehension.'

'He agreed quite readily to renting it back to me. I'll have to be content with that.'

'Content Beth,' Saxon's voice was filled with disgust. 'I fully intend to have a round with him as soon as he's back. I can't wait to knock him down. He's a bounder. How dare he treat you like this, my family are still up in arms about it. Father's tried to talk to the squire but he's not up to it yet.'

Elizabeth squeezed his arm. 'There's nothing we can do Saxon. Our family solicitor, my cousin and I, have all tried. The property is legitimately his now.' She shivered. 'He's more than a bounder, he's cruel and... wicked. You don't know the half of it.' She felt Saxon tense.

'I'll thrash him,' he said.

'Darling Saxon, I wouldn't want to think of you near him, he's too despicable.'

'You wait and see, I'm telling you that I'll have him. He won't be away forever.'

'Saxon please, don't spoil today, it's such a treat to see you, oh I know we write and I value that, but it's not the same as being with you. Do you know, I was coming to see you and your family tomorrow before we go back. I still shall, though it's so good to see you today as well,' she said, smiling up at him.

'I won't be there tomorrow Beth. I've joined up.'

Elizabeth felt as though her heart had stopped beating, her face blanched as she turned to face him, her eyes huge with fear. She gripped his forearms in her hands, holding him secure, as if trying to root him to that spot in Earth Lane. 'No, no Saxon, not you. You can't, I won't let you, do you hear?' She shook him, 'I won't let you.'

He stared at her taken aback by her reaction, as she carried on, her eyes filling with tears. 'Your people, the farm.'

'I know, I've given it a lot of thought, believe me.' Her distress filled him with tenderness and she always seemed to him to be so much smaller when she was off a horse.

'Things don't look so good Beth, I can't stay at home at a time like this and neither can Edward, he's already enlisted.'

'O God, your poor parents,' she released his arms and he drew her into a bear hug, stroking the top of her head clumsily.

'It's all so futile, don't you see Saxon? The best of our young men with their lives before them, sent to fight the same young men of other countries until they're dead or mutilated. Victoria writes to me often and I have insisted that she sends me the parish bulletins. I know of the horrific casualties and losses in this parish alone and it's the same all over the country. Simon Lock missing, Reverend and Mrs. Lock's only son. O God, it's so wicked. Pope Benedict said at the beginning that he would willingly lay down his life if he could only stop this terrible war.' She pressed her face against his chest, the rough tweed of his coat scratched at her as she began to cry uncontrollably.

Saxon felt mortified with the knowledge that he was the cause of her distress, he had no sisters, neither had he any idea how to cope with the situation and was therefore obliged to rely on instinct and his instinct told him to let her sob, releasing the grief she had stored for so long. He continued to hold her close against him, feeling her racking sobs through his body and it was as if all the sadness which she had endured, had now culminated with his announcement.

How long they stood in the lane, wrapped together, he couldn't guess, but eventually her sobs changed into shuddering breaths and she trembled with the aftermath of her outburst. He led her gently to a fallen tree and sat beside her on its trunk, taking a white handkerchief out of his pocket and giving it to her.

'They say that the war won't last long for much longer. I'll tell you what we'll do Beth. When it's all over, we'll meet up here in this spot, under these very trees and think back to today.' He lifted her chin with his hand. 'Promise me?'

She managed a watery smile, 'I promise you.'

He put out his hand. 'Best friends again?'

'My dearest friend in the whole world.'

'And you'll keep writing to me?'

'Of course I will.' She wiped her eyes and face, clutching his handkerchief in her hands.

'We've had some happy times, haven't we Saxon?'

He laughed with a feeling relief that she was calming down, this was more like the Elizabeth he knew. He slapped his thigh, 'Remember out hunting once when we were what, you about nine and me elevenish and we saw those sheepdog puppies at a farm Coxbench way and stopped off to be with them and the field had all gone on ahead and we had no idea where to find them?'

'We went back to the farm to see if they could help us and the farmer's wife made us mugs of cocoa and pointed out the way to the road home.'

'I was punished by my father for being irresponsible.'

'And we found Tom and James on the road home, out looking for us.'

'Aye, we shared a lot of good times with James, I wonder how he's going on? South Notts. Hussars isn't it?'

'Yes,' she stared down at the crisp white edged leaves by her feet.

'Most of them were at Gallipoli, God help them. Do you hear from him?'

'Tom and Annie do, I'm sure he's alright or I'd know.' Her voice was barely audible. They fell silent and he glanced at her and was concerned to see more tears rolling down her face.

'Oh Beth, I'm sorry, I'm such an insensitive fool. When will I ever learn, why you and James were like brother and sister.'

She continued to stare down at the frosted leaves, saying quietly, 'No, Saxon, not at all like brother and sister.'

He looked at her incredulously. 'You're in love with him, with James. Well, I'll be damned.'

She nodded miserably. Something in her expression took his thoughts back to the summer's day before the war, when he had not understood her confusion, try though he had. Now he knew. It all fitted together, how she had coped with so much grief, almost beyond human endurance, she'd had more than family and friends to support her, she'd had someone even closer. Saxon felt as though he had matured in the revelation, as if he now fully understood her.

'What's it like Beth, to be in love?'

She looked up at him, her eyes wide and moist. 'Oh Saxon, it's like being struck by a thunderbolt, like being in heaven, like becoming whole.'

'I didn't realise it could be like that.'

'Oh yes, it came out of the blue, one day we saw each other as if for the first time although we had grown up together.'

'My goodness - do you think it will ever happen to me? I mean when I feel ready for it,' he added self consciously.

'I'm sure it will Saxon. It may start as friendship or it may hit you hard one day, just like that.'

'Could it have happened to us?'

'I suppose it could have done, but we're still at the friendship stage so maybe it wasn't to be.'

He thought this over for a while, then, 'I've made you cry, by reminding you that he's away?'

'I'm crying, not just because he went away, but because he went away from me, you see he left me without a word or a goodbye.'

He felt his heart twist for her whilst he watched helplessly as she began to cry again, though quite calmly now with a kind of wretched finality.

'Why?'

'I don't know. I've racked myself night and day for any possible reason, but I can't find one.' She wiped her face adding miserably. 'He couldn't have loved me, could he?' Her eyes spilling with tears met his. 'Could he?'

He bit his lip feeling out of his depth. 'You can't think that, he must have had his reasons.'

'What possible reason could he have had, to be exactly the same the night before and then to leave so... cruelly. He couldn't have loved me after all.'

She wiped her eyes and then reached for his hand. 'Do you know Saxon, I have never spoken of this to anyone. It says a lot for our friendship that I can tell you, though not much of me to burden you at such a time. I had no intention of doing so, please believe me.'

'Beth, you can't realise how I value you feeling able to confide in me. Goodness knows if you can't talk to me who can you talk to.' His forehead creased. 'Have you not written to each other?'

'I've written dozens of letters and ended up burning them. I did send one letter at the beginning, quite cautiously worded, but he never replied.'

Saxon shook his head, 'I can't believe it. I'm so damned sorry.'

He stood up pulling her to her feet. 'Come on, let's walk back to the house and have some of Mrs. Bailey's cake and tea whilst we thaw out. Who knows, when we keep our rendezvous here after the war everything could have resolved itself, life takes some strange turns Beth.'

Walking back to the farm later, Saxon was able to let his thoughts have free rein. Each day, he and his family scoured the newspapers and parish bulletins and had been horrified at the losses and casualties at Gallipoli, fearing for the Yeomanry Regiments who had been thrown into what had become the last battle there and were still fighting across the Middle East. If the worst came to the worst with James and he didn't, God forbid, make it, or if he really had finished with Beth for whatever reason, then he would take care of her, be there for her. If she wanted marriage, he could see no reason why not, if she'd have him.

He remembered having told her as much before, to her amusement. This resolved, he strode purposefully in the direction of the farm to finish his preparations for leaving.

❧ ❧ ❧

Two days later, before returning to Lincoln, Elizabeth was having afternoon tea with Annie in the parlour of the cottage.

'You're very formal today Annie,' she smiled, taking a slice of treacle tart from a stand.

'You're a young lady now Elizabeth, not the child who sat with us at the kitchen table.'

Elizabeth looked at her slighty startled, 'I hope I'll always be that child to you Annie.'

'Well, you will,' Annie began to laugh, 'I wanted to make an effort for you that's all. It's so nice to see you.'

Elizabeth lay her head back on the comfortably upholstered armchair. 'It's lovely to see you too Annie, I was saying to Saxon a couple of days ago, that no amount of writing can ever compensate for seeing someone.'

'Aye, James said as much in his last letter.' Annie rose and pulled an envelope from behind the clock on the mantle.

Elizabeth moved further forward in her seat. 'How is he Annie, he's alright isn't he?'

'He was, thank God when he sent this this.' Annie passed the letter to her.

Elizabeth held it in her hands. 'May I?'

'Of course.'

Elizabeth felt her heart leap as she saw James' large clear hand-writing. She could hardly read the letter, her eyes had filled with tears, she saw snatches, 'all is well with me... think about you a lot of the time... of all you've done for me... after the war it will be a different world... different values... take good care of each other... God bless you both...'

No mention of her, the stud, the horses, their lives. She became aware of what Annie was saying.

'How I wish he hadn't joined up. Whatever made him do such a thing and at his age too? I've asked myself over and over, why?'

Elizabeth watched her miserably, 'I don't know Annie, I wish I did.'

'Funny, you would have done at one time, you were so close as children and up to James leaving I thought. We must have been mistaken. I suppose as you've grown older, you've grown away from each other. Probably that was to be, but you used to work together so well.'

'Oh Annie,' Elizabeth dashed away the tears which had spilt down her cheeks, 'Annie... Promise you'll write to me and let me know how you both are and how James is?'

'Aye, I will.'

'And the dogs?'

'Aye.'

Elizabeth rose and hugged the person she had known all her life and was one of the closest to her beloved James, 'I shall miss you dearest Annie,' then with a sob, let herself out of the door.

Annie replaced the letter with a sigh. Why James and Elizabeth didn't write to each other was indeed a mystery to her. Maybe, it was that they had just grown apart, but surely even old friends write in wartime?

XVIII

Contrary to James' steadfast refusal to think of Elizabeth or his past life, Elizabeth did little else. For most of her waking hours she dwelt on what had been between them, of his love and support through her darkest days. These thoughts were so tangible that on occasions she felt she could reach out to him. Then would come the dreadful shock of reality, panic at the appaling danger he was in. She prayed for him constantly and vowed to Almighty God that if he could only be spared this terrible conflict, she would, for the rest of her days, bear him no ill-will over his treatment of her.

Her favourite time for reminiscing was during the early hours of the mornings when she was not on duty at Collingswell Hall, a large ancestral home on the outskirts of the city, commandeered by the military as a hospital. Here she worked as a volunteer, performing her duties diligently, whether carrying out menial tasks for the patients, pushing wheelchairs around the grounds, reading or writing their letters. Usually her thoughts were confined to her relationship with James from June 1914, but perversely on this particular morning she was re-living a memory some months previous to that, the 1913 Boxing Day meet of Oakley hounds.

She remembered how cold her fingers had been as she stood on a box, plaiting the mane of Aishling, one of the four-year-olds that she and James had been mainly responsible for breaking in and schooling. The recollection was becoming so real that she could almost smell the young mare and feel the coarse texture of her mane. She hardly dare breathe lest she disturb the magic of her reverie, even to the sound of their voices.

'Tom,' she called through to the neighbouring loosebox, 'will you plait Ashling's tail for me, I'll do the manes, but I never seen to get the tail plaiting tight enough.'

'I'm sure that's not so, but I'll do the tails if you prefer.'

She smiled to herself as she worked, no one, she knew, could plait like Tom, he could make the top of a tail look like sculpture. From the box the other side of her she heard amusement in James' voice. 'Will you do my horses' tails for me as well Pa, I'm not so good at it either.'

'You young scoundrel, you can plait every bit as well as me, the same as Elizabeth can, but she's much more clever at getting her own way.'

'Don't we know it,' James laughed through a length of thread he held between his teeth.

She wove the bodkin into her jersey and pushed the metal comb and thread further into the pocket of her breeches, 'I'll plait two more manes and then I'm going in to have breakfast and change, it wouldn't be good form to be late considering that we only have to ride up to the hall.'

In little over half an hour, transformed, she returned to the yard wearing a dark blue habit with the colour of the Oakley hunt on the collar of her jacket, white stock and top hat with veil. Her father and James were in the stables whilst Tom was rallying two of the stable lads who were to ride second horses along with him.

Elizabeth opened her eyes for a moment as shafts of light began to penetrate the floral curtains in the pretty Edwardian bedroom and then closed them tightly, eager to return to the dream world which held more reality for her...

Once mounted and prepared to leave, she looked up to a window overlooking the yard, hoping her mother would feel well enough to wave them off as she liked to do. Mary didn't disappoint her and her smile held its usual sweetness and warmth. At the kitchen window below, Mrs. Bailey and Jenna waved to them as was also their custom on hunting mornings.

Once on the road, they fell into twos, John and Tom leading,

James and herself following and the lads bringing up the rear.

She glanced down at the mare she rode, noting with satisfaction the immaculate plaits, interested pricked ears and well groomed coat and knew there would be none fitter, better turned out or prepared for the field, than the O'Malley horses.

They passed through the hall gates along with spectators and those who had turned out to follow on foot, whilst on the forecourt, quite a crowd had gathered waiting patiently amongst the horses and riders for hounds to make an appearance. She spotted Saxon Brown on Dolomite. He was talking to the Burdettes, Victoria and her father. He raised his hat with exaggerated courteously and beckoned her over.

'Morning Elizabeth,' he called as she approached, 'horses do you credit.'

She acknowledged the compliment with a smile, then greeted Mr. Burdette and Victoria, the latter mounted on a well bred dappled grey, which she recognised as an O'Malley. Victoria's habit, she noted, was a soft shade of dark grey which flattered the girl's pale complexion and fair hair.

'Lovely morning Elizabeth,' Victoria began, 'as good as a December day could be, perfect going. Oh...' Victoria blushed as she glanced ahead, 'here's Wobert, my, how handsome he looks.'

Robert touched his hat to the group. 'Good morning. As you know my father loves a dramatic entrance, therefore may I wait for the master in such charming company?' Saxon caught her glance and rolled up his eyes.

The atmosphere was broken by an outbreak of cheers as Ralph Oakley, Master of Oakley hounds, made his appearance. Hounds, sterns waving, streamed behind him, held in check by the huntsman and whippers-in, yet managing to take a tit bit from a child in passing or allowing their domed heads to be stroked. The men raised their hats to the master whilst the ladies smiled and nodded and servants from the hall appeared as if by magic with trays of stirrup cups and small savouries.

Robert handed glasses to the girls, 'I'm saving you from a fate worse than death,' he said, jerking his head in Saxon's direction. 'Whatever you do, never accept a drink from our friend here, not unless you want to be sticking to cherry brandy on your horse's neck all day.' He turned sharply to the footman. 'Fetch me a man's drink, a large one. Whisky for you eh Saxon?'

'No, really thanks, a sherry will do me fine, anything stronger at this time of day and I'll disappear over the horizon never to be seen again.'

'We live in bloody hopes,' Robert muttered irritably under his breath, then snatching a chunky glass from the returning footman, pushed him back with his booted toe. 'Took your bloody time didn't you?'

Elizabeth felt her face flush with disgust as she recalled his ill humour and opening her eyes was disorientated for a moment. She closed them quickly and was immediately transported back to her memories of that day...

She excused herself and rode over to her father who was talking to the squire. Ralph raised his cap to her. 'Morning Elizabeth, I trust you've had a good Christmas?'

'Lovely, master, thank you, and you?'

'Ups and downs m'dear, ups and downs.' He grimaced amusingly then touched his hat with his crop and turned to a group beside them.

'Ralph tells me we're going to draw Holly Copse first and then on to the coverts at Derwent Farm,' John informed her. 'I'll ask Tom to have the second horses down at the farm for lunch time.'

She nodded as one of the whippers in began to call up stray hounds, cracking his whip above the heads of the renegades. 'Come up, Rattler, Royston, Vanquish.' He cracked his whip again as they loped off towards the rest of the pack. 'Hold to.'

She watched one of her favourite sights, hounds flowing like a torrent, master, huntsmen and whippers-in, in their red coats with the brass buttons of the hunt. She fell in with the field behind them, sensing the interest of the young horse beneath her and its anticipation of its first day out with hounds.

She could hear Sarah, her aunt's maid outside the bedroom door, clattering the tea tray as she balanced it on her knee whilst she knocked. Elizabeth glanced around the room with a slight feeling of guilt, had anything been left of that day to betray her absence from the present time? How ridiculous, she chided herself, calling to the girl to come in.

The day passed slowly, Elizabeth went for a walk, exploring the secret ways of Lincoln with which her aunt's brother-in-law, Wilfred, had acquainted her. On her days off, she alternated her walks, sometimes down Steep Hill past the Jews House and on into the town, other times she would walk as far as the Ermine, returning back cold and glowing, to tea and crumpets in front of the fire with her aunt, thawing out her toes and fingers to enable her to write letters, or knit and sew the khaki comforts for the troops which her aunt had volunteered for the ladies circle at the Catholic Church of St. Hugh on Monks Road. It was at this church that she attended Mass with her aunt, lit candles and said her Rosary, beseeching the intercession of the Holy Mother and St. James for James' and Saxon's safety. She spent much of her off duty hours writing to Saxon, Annie, Victoria and her old friend Florence in Nottingham, with whom she had attended Catechism classes along with James.

Elizabeth retired early and disciplined herself to sleep so that she could have an early start transporting herself back to that Boxing day meet, which during the daytime seemed so long ago...

They rode across a couple of fields to the dark mass of Holly Copse, foot followers opening and closing gates for them at this stage. The huntsman had already put hounds in and their voices could be heard as they worked amongst the dead bracken and cover. She and her father positioned themselves down wind of the copse and waited quietly with the rest of the field although they couldn't see James. Probably at the side of the covert, he'd more sense than to wait upwind, she concluded as she listened to the familiar comments being hoarsely whispered by a few locals around them, snatches of which reached her ears.

'I 'ope they have a good day, that old dog fox is killing a dozen or more fowls every week, often in daylight he's become so bold. No matter how well they're shut up he'll burrow under the wire else squeeze through a gap seemingly not two inches wide.'

His companion nodded sagely and took up the narrative. 'He'll be the one that had my wife's geese only last week, our Christmas dinner and the rest of the family's. We give some as gifts you see. She broke her heart I can tell you, the damned thing took one and left five others mauled and mutilated, one of the farm workers left the barn door a crack but that's enough for them buggers.' He caught her eye. 'You'll pardon me miss.'

Smoke hung in the air from the second man's pipe, she wanted to ask him not to smoke or for that matter to talk whilst hounds were working, but felt it would be churlish to do so. She needn't have worried, a brown shape slid out of the undergrowth, she heard the 'view holloa' called from several quarters before hounds streamed out of the copse, under and over the post and rail fence and pursued the fox down towards the valley. Hounds were now in full cry, their crashing music echoing around the hill. The cold rush of air in her face, plough and grass land lit with the pale rays of the winter sun, the smell of disturbed earth were adrenaline to her as she let the young mare give of her best. She saw the first flight take a wide thorn hedge and set Aishling directly at it. The mare needed no urging, taking off exactly when she asked and as they flew over the top she found another rider by her side who had jumped simultaneously and saw it was James, giving his four-year-old its head. She squinted her eyes across the other riders searching for her father, spotting him in mid jump and saw with satisfaction that the youngster he was riding was going well.

Hounds slowed up by Low Wood, deep in the valley, working the dense undergrowth, releasing the scent of trampled leaves and mould. They had lost him. There were other good runs that day, but the old dog fox evaded the hunt yet again and darkness threatened. Riding home the second horses which they had exchanged at lunch time, their original ones hacked home by Tom and the lads, John opened a packet of bacon sandwiches which he had saved from lunch.

She laughed joyously. 'Oh Papa how funny, less than a mile away and you've saved those as we do on longer rides home.'

'And, not only these but a flask of port too my dear, you may well laugh, but these kind of habits are tradition and the ride home, long or short couldn't possibly be the same without them.' He passed the flask to her and she to James before John emptied it and wiped his mouth with the back of his hand. 'There now, we're properly fortified,' he said as they rode the short distance to the stud.

Elizabeth found herself smiling, she had felt so close to Papa and was reluctant to open her eyes. How she wished she could stay in that safe, happy world and not return. Almost immediately she felt ashamed of her thoughts. No one could have been kinder than Aunt Martha who had so much of her mother's gentle nature that Elizabeth found great comfort in her company. Just returning in spirit to those days would suffice for now, she decided, and for the rest, time alone would prove.

XIX

1918

The long drawn out fight against the Turkish Army took James' regiment the length and breadth of Palestine. The Yeomanry Regiments and their horses, mules and donkeys, suffered deaths, casualties, disease, thirst and hunger. By March 1918 the Turkish Armies were broken, the Yeomanry had done their job and the British Armies in France were in need of more troops.

On 2nd April, the South Notts. Hussars paraded for the last time as cavalry. Horses and saddlery were handed to the Remount Depot at Belah and the regiment, retaining only the Hotchkiss gun and personal equipment, became part of the Warwick and South Notts. Machine Gun Battalion.

After dark on the 26th May, the battalion set sail for France on the *Leasowe Castle*, as one of a convoy of six transports, accompanied by destroyers, trawlers, aeroplanes and a captive kite balloon. The men had been ordered to sleep on deck in their emergency positions. James' detail included Toby Mallett and Harry Brown. The night was bright with moonlight and although circled by the flotilla, the men were on edge.

'By God we're standing out like sore thumbs. Why are we sailing tonight of all nights? It's damned nearly as light as day.' Toby's whisper was tense, 'I hate the bloody sea. I'm beginning to feel churned up inside already. All I can do about it is keep still, suffer and pray it will soon be over.' He rubbed his hand over his face anxiously. 'Will it take us long Jim, this sailing?'

James tried to reassure him, cajole him, as had become his habit since Toby had suffered more and more from nerves and shell shock.

'At the moment Tobe, the priority is to get as much sea behind us as possible. Give it another hour and we should be out of harm's way.'

'God willing,' Harry said through an unlit cigarette in his mouth. 'We're under strict orders to keep all lights out yet we're sailing in this bloody spotlight, might as well be on stage.' He pocketed his cigarette with reluctance.

'Aye, making our names,' James said dryly. 'Come on, let's get some rest.' Rest didn't come easily though, and they continued to speak quietly and intermittently until after midnight.

Toby held his stomach. 'Oh God, it's getting worse. I feel awful. They say you're not so bad at night, when you can't see anything that is. Some hopes on a night like this.' He slid down into a reclining position. 'But then, I don't have to see the bloody swell to feel it.' He was restless for a while and then suddenly leapt up and rushed to the side of the ship, to vomit overboard.

'Good job you're down wind Toby,' a voice close to him whispered hoarsely. 'Make sure you keep it that way, else you'll be popular.' One or two stifled laughs followed.

James shook his head to Harry. 'Poor sod.' He made way as Toby dropped down beside him. He could hear Toby's teeth chattering and feel him shivering. 'Where's your canteen? Try a swallow of water.'

Toby shook his head.

'Come on, it'll make you feel better.' Toby did as he was bid, like an obedient child, James thought, with sadness.

'There are rumours going round that we might get some home leave when the battalion reaches France,' Harry whispered. 'Them of us who have been out here for so long, that is. See my wife and kids.' He smiled at the thought. 'How about that then Toby?'

'I'd sooner see my Ma and sisters,' Toby muttered, with a half hearted attempt at humour. Who do you most want to see Jim?'

'Ma and Pa.'

'Have you got a girl?'

'No.'

'Have you ever had a girl? I mean apart from the one you met in Nottingham that night and the odd ones we've chatted up since,' Toby persevered.

Toby didn't usually pry, James thought, for they had all long since accepted James' reticence to discuss his business.

James looked out to sea, watching the rise and fall of the waves, then down at the deck. 'I once thought I had,' he said quietly.

They fell silent.

Harry yawned. 'We should be a fair way out to sea by now,' he commented, taking out his watch. 'Let's try for some shut eye, it's way past midnight.'

❧ ❧ ❧

They had scarcely closed their eyes in an uneasy attempt at sleep, when a torpedo hit the *Leasowe Castle* amidships, on the starboard side. James felt himself catapulted into a group of men behind him who were struggling to their feet, the sickening crash of the impact temporarily deafening him. In the seconds it took to recover himself, he became aware that the engines had stopped, the pulsing life of the ship stilled. Although voices could be heard from all directions, James was impressed by the calmness which prevailed, for no one was more aware than he that although these men had just about seen it all, they were none of them seamen. He glanced round relieved to see Harry helping Toby to his feet.

The troops paraded at their stations as rolls were called, boats lowered and rafts thrown overboard. A Japanese destroyer stood by, whilst the rest of the convoy continued on their way at full speed and rapidly disappeared.

James, Toby and Harry, helped lower some of the forty life boats whilst the *Leasowe Castle* remained on a fairly even keel, though sinking a little at the stern with a slight list to port. All of 'B' Warwickshire Yeomanry Company of the battalion went over the port side and were picked up in the water.

James saw Toby watching them forlornly, whilst continuing to help lower the remaining boats into the sea. In the moonlight, he could see that Toby's face was deadly pale and that he was suffering from the shakes. He slapped Toby on the back. 'Soon be our turn Tobe, we're doing alright.'

The Japanese vessel had put up a smoke screen. Harry peered through it. 'The cavalry's here, thank God,' he said, pointing to a sloop on its way back to them from the convoy. As she got nearer, they could make out her name, *H.M. Lily*. She ran her bows along the starboard bow of the *Leasowe Castle* and made fast, so that some of the troops were able to pass quickly on board.

Suddenly, around two in the morning a bulkhead in the aft part of the ship gave way and with a loud rending noise the *Leasowe Castle* sank rapidly by the stern, the bows rearing straight on end. The *Lily* had a narrow escape, as the hawsers connecting her with the sinking ship were cut with an axe only at the very last minute.

James, Harry and Toby along with scores of other men still on board, slid down the part of the deck yet unsubmerged, battered against each other and objects on deck, before being shot into the sea. James felt the tremendous suction as the ship went down and he with it, terrifyingly aware that the air not knocked from his lungs by the hammering slide down the deck was now being squeezed from his chest by his rapid plunge under the water. He fought against the descent, willing his legs to push him upwards, or what he hoped was upwards, through the total blackness. Water filled his nostrils and mouth, threatening to choke him and again he tried to force his legs to push him up. His efforts were totally ineffectual.

Panic seized him as he felt himself being dragged even further down with the ship. *This is it,* he thought. *I haven't really cared whether I make it or not, yet now the time has come, I don't want to die this way, not by the sea.* He became aware of the medallion of St. James, which had risen under his chin. *Saint James, help me.* A third time he struggled, giving it all he had, pushing with his legs whilst he fought to hold his breath. His protesting lungs felt as though they would burst, forcing him to open his mouth in an effort to breathe, taking in a volume of sea water. His head became water-logged, whilst his legs took on weight and his whole body began to feel leaden. *Saint James, help me.* He made a gargantuan effort.

Above him the uncompromising blackness turned grey and then lighter grey as he surfaced into the moonlight. The sea was bubbling with men, struggling like him to keep afloat. He trod water, coughing and spluttering, whilst he gulped air. He caught a piece of wreckage and clung to it whilst he continued to cough and retch. Heads were bobbing all around him, struggling to get onto the rafts, hands reaching out. James felt someone grab the back of his tunic and pull him over the side, he lay for a moment conscious of rough boards beneath his cheek. He dragged himself to a sitting position and was appalled by the weight of his sodden uniform which caused his movements to be slow and cumbersome. *How had he made it to the surface?* He felt for the medallion and clutching it, made a silent prayer to his patron saint.

'Toby?' he looked around at the men on the raft. 'Have any of you seen Toby Mallett?'

They shook their heads.

'Harry Brown?' No one spoke. James closed his eyes and dropped his head, water swilled in his ears and through it he heard muffled sounds, the slap of water on the edge of the raft, the shouts of men being pulled from the sea, the groans of the injured, seemingly a long way away, until he could hear them no more.

The survivors were taken from the rafts and into rowing boats. James was hardly aware of the change over, he had never felt so completely exhausted in his life. His heavy wet uniform clung to his body, icy cold, his throat felt raw and the taste of salt water was in his nose and mouth. From time to time, he trembled, uncontrollably. The sea was calm except for a slight swell but many of the men were seasick. James watched them with a heavy heart, picturing Toby not so long before in the same plight. His throat constricted, he put his head in his arms and endured the long, long night.

Dawn broke eventually. James and his fellow survivors watched the injured being taken aboard the Japanese ship. As rowing boats passed them, a trooper called to James, 'Gretton, Harry Brown's been asking after you.'

'He made it?' James tried to shout but his voice had almost gone.

'He's injured, not badly he should be alright, he was one of the first aboard the Jap ship, I'll tell him I've seen you. Good luck mate.'

'Toby Mallett?' James croaked, but the man was out of earshot, pulling on the oars, heading for the ship.

By mid-morning rescue ships arrived and took James and the remaining survivors to Alexandria, arriving at 7pm on the 27th May. Although the survivors were in bad shape, at least James thought, they were alive. It was when he was at the height of a raging cold and fever, he learned that 50 men of the South Notts., who had gone down with the *Leasowe Castle* had not been recovered. Toby, with his terrible fear of the sea, was amongst them.

⚜ ⚜ ⚜

On the 18th June the battalion set sail once more, this time on *HMT Caledonia* in a convoy consisting of five ships. They reached the Italian Naval port of Taranto on the 23rd June. James and Harry found themselves on a long, slow journey by train, herded in forties with other men, into rail goods vans, which would have made the journey intolerable had it not been for frequent halts and the fine scenery of the east coast of Italy and the French Riviera, skirting Marseilles and Paris, reaching Estaples by 29th June.

The long awaited leave home, commenced.

XX

'You look lovely Elizabeth.' Aunt Martha said admiringly. She stood close by Elizabeth in front of a long mirror, and put her arm across Elizabeth's shoulders. 'I'm so pleased you let me talk you into having such a such a beautiful new outfit made. You're young, you deserve it. Goodness knows, you've scrimped enough along with the rest of us for the war effort.'

Elizabeth kissed her cheek, 'How long did you have this piece of blue silk stacked away aunt?'

'Twenty years at least, my dear. We certainly couldn't have got anything like it now, neither in Lincoln or Nottingham, and I wouldn't hold out too much hope of getting it in London, not without knowing the right people that is. I'm fully aware how it's become almost immoral to dress well these days, but I haven't noticed the Royal family looking exactly impoverished in the photographs which appear of them in the press.' She studied Elizabeth's reflection again with evident pride.

'That chic little hat is perfect, well worth getting Madame Bouverie out of retirement for. Mr. Neeson will hardly recognise you. Such a nice man and he cares for your interests as well as he would his own, I've the highest regard for him.'

'You don't think I look overdressed for a business appointment with Mr. Neeson and a day out in Nottingham?'

'Not at all my dear. He'll be as pleased as punch to see you looking so well and anyhow we're going to make the most of the day, a little shopping and lunch out. Whilst we've been most fortunate that quite often dear Wilfred has taken us over to see Mr. Neeson in his automobile, I really haven't liked to put on him by dawdling in Nottingham as we are able to when travelling by the railway.' She put on her hat, setting it at a somewhat jaunty angle, 'Let's make the most of it today.'

Elizabeth nodded as she pulled on her gloves.

❧ ❧ ❧

For almost four years Elizabeth had seen the terrible influx of injured men who had been shipped home and were being unloaded at the railway stations. She still found the sight as grievous and shocking as she had on the first occasion. At Lincoln St Marks Station, orderlies were carrying stretchers from ambulance trains which had just pulled in. Injured servicemen, some, little more than boys, lay inert, with faces so pale and drained of blood that they looked already dead. Head wounds were commonplace as were men with eyes bandaged, holding onto their colleagues. Her experience at Collingswell Hall, had in no way lessened her horror of the appalling suffering.

As Elizabeth and her aunt disembarked from the train at Nottingham Midland Station, the situation was, if anything, worse. The platforms were full of the injured, most of them stretcher cases. Amongst them men on leave, soldiers, sailors and odd members of the Royal Flying Corps wove their way through, pausing here and there to give a cigarette to one of the wounded, or talk with them. Men stared at her, with eyes that had seen hell, some delirious, garbling, trickles of saliva running from their mouths, their injuries horrific. Limbs amputated, heads and faces burned, torn and mutilated. Some, evidently mistaking Elizabeth and her aunt, for loved ones, reached out to them. In these men, Elizabeth saw James and Saxon and was overcome with compassion. She touched them and forced herself to smile, her lips trembling with emotion.

The walking wounded and men on leave, eyed her up, making admiring comments and one of the more bold tried to walk alongside them and engage Elizabeth in conversation. Despite Aunt Martha taking her arm and steering her away, the man was persistent and Elizabeth cast her eyes downwards. Had Elizabeth not kept her gaze so firmly to the ground, she would have seen a group of South Notts.

Hussars, laughing and talking as they made their way out of the station on their first leave in over three years.

James had just paused to light a cigarette for a stretcher case and exchange a few words, when he looked up and saw Elizabeth and her aunt, walking past. James' eyes were transfixed. His chest tightened and he could hardly draw breath. He felt his throat constrict and it was all he could do to prevent himself from reaching out to her. She passed so close to him that he could smell the fragrance of her. His head became light and swam with memories, her beauty, her passion, all they had shared.

The soldier on the stretcher watched him, 'She's a vision if ever there was one, mate. You've got good taste.' He laughed coarsely and then began to cough, tearing at his lungs, his eyes bulging. 'Gas,' he wheezed, between bouts.

James stayed by him until he quietened, following Elizabeth with his eyes as she clutched her aunt's arm and hurried from the station. Could she have seen him? No, he knew that she hadn't. Her aunt seemed to be getting her away from what looked like a Sherwood Forester who was trying to latch onto them. He watched until they were out of sight, whilst he hung back, ignoring the calls from Harry and the other troopers.

'Come on Jim, we've waited long enough for this, what's keeping you?'

James made his way over to them, 'You go, I'm alright, I'll be waiting for Pa to pick me up.' He slapped their backs, 'Enjoy your leave, every minute of it. God knows we've earned it.' He watched them go off, hurrying to their families, wives and sweethearts.

He waited a little longer, until he was sure that Elizabeth and her aunt had gone, then tentatively made his way out to the front of the station to look for Tom, his mind in turmoil. What if she was going to Oakley? He knew he could not bring himself to go if that was the case. Could the great Captain Oakley be on leave and she was going to see him? He couldn't get over how elegant she looked. That, he thought cynically, was what became of taking up with the son of a rich man, particularly one who had purloined her home and land and was in a position to hold this over her. She didn't look exactly downtrodden though, he reasoned, in fact she looked beautiful, even more so than he remembered. His heart twisted. God help me, he thought in anguish, why did this have to happen?

'James.'

He turned and saw Tom behind him, stepping down from the back of a trap.

'Pa,' James ran to him and embraced him, hugging him tightly, 'Pa, it's so good to see you.'

Tom, his arms around James sniffed back tears, 'Thanks be to God, you're home, my boy, we've missed you more than you'll ever know.' He caught James' arms and held them by his side, 'Here, let me look at you. So much taller than me now, but we'll need to get more flesh on you. Ma will soon see to that. My, but she'll hardly know you.' He steered James towards the trap. 'Come on let's get going, she's cooking something special.'

James hesitated, 'Pa.' Tom looked at him.

'Pa, is there any chance Elizabeth will be at the stud?'

Tom shook his head, 'No James, I'm sorry, but she won't, so don't build your hopes up, she always lets us know when she's coming, usually to do with business.'

'But might she today?' James persisted.

'No. Your Ma and Elizabeth exchanged letters quite recently, just before we knew you were coming home on leave but she didn't mention anything and she would have done.' Tom urged James into the trap, 'She comes to Oakley when we go by the local railway up to Gatthorpe and to Nottingham to see the family solicitor and then goes back to Lincoln.' He wove the trap through hackney carriages, horse drawn ambulances and the odd few motorised ambulances and turned the pony's head towards home.

'That, Ma, was something I've dreamed about for a long time.' James said, putting his knife and fork together on the empty plate.

'There you are you see, the army can't compare with my cooking.' Annie laughed, then more seriously, said, 'You should never have left James, you were only a boy, I'll never understand it.'

James put his hand on her arm, 'One day Ma, I'll tell you, but I can say that my reason was not in any way connected with you or Pa.'

Annie stroked his hair as she passed behind with the plates, 'Well, you're home now, that's all that matters, home where you belong.' She opened the oven door and drew out a fruit pie, golden, with steam rising through the funnel and placed it on the table, then reached to the top of the range for a jug of custard.

James watched her, his eyes moving from her familiar kindly face, to her hands as she cut the pie and served him some, hands that had nurtured him since babyhood, hands into which his dying parents had entrusted him.

✄ ✄ ✄

Just after 7pm as they were relaxing in the parlour, there was an almighty explosion which seemed to rock the house.

Annie blanched, 'Dearest Lord, we're being invaded!'

The three of them ran out of the cottage. Mrs. Bailey was out in the top yard along with Joe and Eddie.

'God help them Annie, it's got to be the bomb factory at Chilwell.'

Everyone's eyes turned to the south west, in the direction of Chilwell, no more than six miles from them, where great clouds of smoke and flames could be seen in the sky.

'Jenna and her sister work there,' Mrs. Bailey wrung her hands in her apron, 'They came to see me only last week. Oh, pray they weren't at work tonight.' She began to sob and Annie put her arms around her and led her to the cottage. The men in the yard were joined by others from the village, all white faced and tight lipped at the horror on their doorstep.

Late afternoon the following day Tom came in with the

Nottingham Evening Post and pointed out a small article in a right hand column.

'Look at this,' he exclaimed in disgust, slapping the paper with the back of his hand, 'That's all that's been reported on an explosion of this proportion.'

Annie and James spread the paper on the table and read the report:

Last night's explosion in Midland Shell Factory. Death Roll of between 60-70. Number of injured not yet known. It went on to describe the bravery of women workers.

'I'll take a bet that there's been reporting restrictions on it,' James said as he studied the article, 'Mrs. Bailey heard a different story from Jenna and her sister this morning.'

Annie nodded, 'Aye, it's a miracle those two are safe, they'd just come off the day shift. They told Mrs. Bailey and Eddie who drove her over, they'd heard this morning that the clock at the factory stopped at twelve minutes past seven, just after the night shift had turned in. That was when the explosion happened.'

'The first of July, two years to the day of the Somme offensive,' James said slowly, 'either an unbelievable coincidence or something else.'

Tom and Annie looked up. 'Sabotage?' they said in union.

James tightened his lips, 'Chances are we'll never know.'

'No more than we'll know how many were really killed and injured.'

'To think that I was planning to try for a job there.'

Tom and Annie stared at him in surprise.

'I left for the Hussars instead.'

'I never thought I would be thankful for that, James,' Annie said with feeling.

They glanced at the minimal article again in disbelief. Below was a lengthy column on the influenza epidemic, reporting an alarming outbreak in a convent at Westminster.

Annie traced the article with her finger, reading aloud: *More deaths reported. The influenza epidemic seems to be spreading with great rapidity.* She glanced at the others, 'It goes from one thing to another doesn't it? When will things ever return to normality?'

'We shall never return to what we knew as normality Ma, too much has happened.' James folded the newspaper.

Tom agreed with him, 'He's right Annie. What with the war and so many tragic events and then of all things John losing the place.'

'What could he have been thinking of?'

Tom covered Annie's hand with his, 'We'll never know what was in his mind, he wasn't himself at all, the poor man had endured so much and in such a short time.'

Annie took a handkerchief out of her pinafore pocket and wiped her eyes, 'I often try to imagine what he suffered knowing that he had gambled Elizabeth's inheritance away? All he had worked for and his family before him.'

Tom sighed, 'Remember that he was drinking heavily at that time and staying up at the hall all hours. There was many a morning I called at the house to see him because he wasn't out in the yard in his usual way.' Tom rubbed his eyes, 'Sometimes he would come out later and be more or less his old self, like when he told me about his plans for the horses and growing animal feedstuff for the army. Damned good idea that's proved to be an' all.'

'Yes I'm sure it is Pa, but for how long? When the war's over that bastard Oakley will soon put a stop to this rented arrangement.

'James, no need to talk like that,' Annie admonished him.

'You don't know what he's like Ma or how I've always felt about him, there are few people I really can't stand but he's one of them. He's got what he wanted now hasn't he? His sort always do.'

'Do you think he wanted this place then, I mean before the card game? I know it's no secret in these parts that one of John's ancestors got it that way, but they were different days weren't they?' She bit her bottom lip, 'Do you think that?' She looked at James anxiously, 'I mean that he'd wanted it all along?'

James was a while before answering. 'Something like that,' he said quietly. They sat in silence for a while, each with their own thoughts. James pulled himself upright in his chair and drummed his fingers on the table, 'I hadn't wanted to broach any of this so soon in my leave, but I suppose now is as good a time as any. I've given a lot of thought to what I want to talk to you about.'

Tom glanced at Annie as they settled down to listen.

'I would like you to look for a place of our own that we can rent. It needn't have much land but it must have a good sized yard and of course a house for us.' He took hold of Annie's hand as she tried to interrupt.

'Make no mistake Ma, when this war is over, Captain Oakley will get rid of us all. He won't want any of John O'Malley Sullivan's people left here.'

'But Elizabeth is renting the place, she wouldn't allow it,' Tom said earnestly, 'I know her better than that.'

'She'll have no say in it, not if she wants to keep it on to rebuild the business.'

'Why should it matter to Captain Oakley who works here, especially as John appointed Tom to manage the business for her?' Annie asked him.

'Remember that she's nearly twenty one.'

'Elizabeth would never let us be treated like that,' Annie said confidently.

'You don't know anyone when their back is to the wall. She'll go along with Oakley...' James paused, 'She already has. What choice did she have if this place was so damned important to her? When all is said and done, it belongs to him, house, stable yards, outbuildings and land.'

'How can you be so sure that Elizabeth has as you say, 'gone along with him'?' Tom asked.

'Because Oakley himself told me,' James said simply.

Tom and Annie looked at him incredulously.

'There seems a lot we don't know about,' Tom said.

James nodded slowly and tightened his lips.

When Tom spoke again, his voice was low, 'What do you propose we'll do with this place you want us to look for?'

'Start up our own business. I've saved the best part of my pay since I joined up. You told me once that my parents had left me a little money for when I reach twenty one, which isn't long now. We'll make out.'

'Doing what?' Tom asked again.

'Motorised livestock transport Pa, that's what. It's the thing of the future, I've thought it all out. Drovers will become obsolete when more automobiles are on the roads. Horses will no longer be moved in wagons pulled by Shires. The railways will still do their share of movement but they can't stand markets and fairs and load up livestock there and then. We could, and what's more we could drive them anywhere, anywhere at all.' James eyes shone with enthusiasm, 'It's the thing of the future Pa and we can be amongst the first.'

'Where would we get a wagon as big and strong as the railway have and who can drive an automobile? I certainly can't.'

'We'll buy a strong lorry chassis and have a wagon built onto it, get a craftsman to do it, a joiner, and have the metal done by a blacksmith. It will be big, strong and safe, we'll see to that and then we'll be in business.' He smiled, 'I'll be driving by then, I promise you.'

Tom rubbed his chin and said thoughtfully, 'It does sound feasible James. It's certainly an idea if the worst comes to the worst and our first loyalty will always lie with you, but you must realise that I am honour bound to John's daughter until she is at least twenty one.'

'I know that Pa, but as I've already said, she'll soon be twenty one and that combined with her affiliation with Captain Oakley, doesn't bode well for you.'

'James, how can we leave Elizabeth, after all that's happened? We'd have to be convinced that she didn't need us anymore. Then to leave this house, Pa and me have been here since we got married. All these years...' Annie's voice was tremulous

'I know Ma, and I understand what it means to you, but things aren't the same and never will be again. I won't stand by and see you thrown out. Listen to me and let's have our own place before that happens. There's got to be smallholdings, that kind of thing standing empty. Let's look around and find something suitable.'

'But Pa has always worked with stock.'

'If we have a bit of land we can get some stock of our own, but in any case livestock transporters need experience with stock, they wouldn't be much good without now would they?'

Annie shook her head.

'Whilst I'm on leave I'll look around, see what there is going, at least get some idea, though what I really want is for both of you to like a new place, get the feel of it and see if you could settle there.'

'Let's sleep on it lad. It's all come as a bit of a shock to us. Give us time.'

X X 1

1918

It was in July that Marshall Foch commenced his plans for the great allied counter attack. The first move was made by French and American troops on the Marne. On 8th August an offensive was launched on the line from Morlancourt, north of the Somme to Brasches on the Avre, by the Fourth Army and French First Army. The enemy were driven back from their position near Amiens, in five days the Fourth Army captured 400 guns and around 22,000 prisoners.

On 21st August a further attack was made by the Third and Fourth Armies, when the town of Albert was taken and by the end of the month the entire line from Arras to Soissons was steadily advancing. By 1st September, Amiens had been disengaged, Bapaume taken and the Battle of the Scarpe compelled the enemy to withdraw to the Tortille River and the Nurlu Plateau in front of the Hindenburg Line.

It was at this stage that the South Notts. and Warwickshire Battalion began to take an active part in these operations. Orders were received for the battalion to march fifteen miles to Trones Wood. The route lay through the heart of the devastated area by Albert and through the valley of the Ancre. Everywhere was pitted with shell holes. Past Fricourt, Mametz and Montaunban, places which were to become famous in the history of the war, but were now mere masses of debris. The battalion passed the Chateau of Baycourt, near Albert, which by some chance was left standing and was being used as Divisional Headquarters.

On 16th September the Third Army Corps commenced an attack on the whole front, with the object of breaking through the Hindenburg line by taking Epehy, the South Notts. coming for a time under the orders of the 18th Machine Gun Battalion. On the 17th an initial covering barrage was put up, the guns being laid by compass, as all fire was indirect, the same procedure being carried out the following day. Fifteen thousand rounds were fired by the South Notts. on the 19th in support of the infantry attack The battalion was again in action on the 21st sustaining fourteen wounded. James Gretton was amongst them.

✂ ✂ ✂

James lay in a pool of blood, although semi-conscious he could feel the searing pain in his left leg where the shell had torn through to the bone. He tried to moisten his lips but his tongue felt as dry as a rasp. His head hurt, he could feel the warm cloying stickiness of blood seeping over his face. There were explosions all around him and he pressed his face further into the ravaged earth. Where there were seconds between shelling, he could hear the cries and moans of the wounded. This, he thought with finality, is the end of it all. His mind slipped into the void between consciousness.

The deaths of Joe and Fred, Toby and so many others... screams of the wounded being burned alive... Ron Shelton missing at Gallipoli, never heard of again... men and horses dying of thirst and exhaustion in the arid wastes of Palestine... horses, trudging over hills for two days under a blazing sun with neither food nor drink... the Turks burned our grain... horses falling as they took their final breath, eyes open, bulging with the effort they had made. Shells, eternal shells. Horses tied up to rails, terrified by the shelling, kicking the horses beside them to pulp... couldn't get away... tied fast. Heads, mere cavities, men and horses alike, brains blown out of them... limbs scattered... bones shattered... intestines spilled. He'd seen it all... now it was his turn. Been home, told Ma and Pa to find somewhere, thank God, couldn't have them thrown out. Saw Beth, saw her for the last time, could have reached out to her, could have touched her... one last time...

Bright moon through the haze of smoke, was this death? Always a bright moon, Toby drowned in a bright moon. Tried to look after him. Visited Toby's Ma... Toby had called out for his Ma... was to be, getting leave, tied up the ends. It was to be.

His eyes were open but he couldn't see the moonlight anymore.

XXII

James could hear quiet voices moving amongst the fallen around him. 'Over here George, there's one alive, but only just by the looks of him.'

James didn't know who they were talking about. When they put their hands on him he could have screamed aloud yet some instinct made him bite back the sound as they lifted him onto a stretcher and carried him away at a semi-jog. Pain from his leg shot through his nerves like red hot wires and his head felt it was about to burst.

He thought, *Oh God, let me die. I'd far rather had not been moved, left to die in preference to this torture. They know not what they do. He'd heard these words many times before, where he wondered? Why were they so poignant now? Perhaps his mind had gone and if, God forbid, he recovered, he would be brain damaged, a nervous wreck, shell shocked beyond any hope of recovery.*

'Leave me, please leave me to die with the rest, I could bear the pain lying close to the earth, but not now, not now...' his mouth moved but the words were silent, indecipherable. He tried to swallow, get control of his speech, but his dry, swollen tongue seemed to fill his mouth. 'Take someone who can be saved, put me back on the ground for mercies sake.' The laboured words were no more coherent than his first attempt. He shut his eyes and gritted his teeth against the jolting torment as the jogging continued, occasionally rocking him from side to side, loosing silent screams from within him.

❧ ❧ ❧

Somewhere in the strange plateau of returning consciousness he heard the sound of water being poured. He moved his head in the direction of the sound and tried to open his eyes but they seemed to be covered with something. He was filled with panic and moved his right hand up to his face and began to pluck at bandages which covered his head. He heard a voice, which seemed very distant and felt a hand take hold of his, restraining his efforts to loose the bandage.

'There now my dear, you're back in the land of the living, thank God.' The voice spoke English and he relaxed his spine.

'Where am I?' The words were hoarse and hardly audible.

'You're in a hospital, safe.' The pressure of the hand increased a little.

'Who are you?'

'A nurse, your nurse.'

'Am I blind?'

'Well now, we shall soon be knowing when the medical officer hears of you regaining consciousness.'

He tried to pull his hand free, desperate to take off the restraining cloth.

'No, no, no. If you promise to leave the bandage where it is, I'll go and find the doctor, but first I must have your promise.'

'Don't be long.'

'I did say your promise.'

'Alright, but please don't be long.' He felt her release his hand and sensed her turning away, hearing the rustle of what he imagined to be her starched apron.

His thoughts ran riot. If he had lost his sight, when would it have been? He strove to remember falling in battle, but couldn't. All he could remember was the hopelessness and what he had considered to be his final despair. How could he take stock of his injuries? He only knew that he hurt all over. Tentatively he began to examine himself. He knew, at least, that apart from feeling leaden and aching, there was nothing wrong with his right arm. He moved his left arm and curled his fingers, the joints felt stiff and heavy but by the exploration of his right hand he knew that the limb was there. He moved the toes of his right leg and bent his knee fractionally, it felt the same as his arms, yet intact.

A little more confident now, he tried the same with his left leg. Pain burst like a bomb and then his head seemed to turn to ice as he remembered hearing that amputees could still feel pain in a limb after it had been amputated. He reached his left arm down to the leg and felt what seemed like boards and bindings, but he could not feel the limb. He lay back motionless, his thoughts in turmoil. *Damn them, how soon would they tell him the extent of his injuries. Blind with one leg, God, how could he cope with it?* Yet he knew that thousands were already having to do so, both allies and enemy alike. He did not pursue the investigation of his face and head for he had given his word, but the possibility of blindness terrified him. *Perhaps,* he thought, *if his sight were spared he could learn to manage with no left leg. Would he ever be able to ride again?*

Perversely, he had never thought of disabling injuries, only of life and death, one or the other, no middle course, no second chance. *What chance,* he thought, *now, if I'm blind. Never again to see the white blossom of the thorn hedges in England, the swallows coming home, see the skylarks rising higher and higher as they sang.* Tears filled his eyes. *Could a blind man cry? Of course they could.* He tried to control it, but the hot tears spilled into his lashes which felt stiff and hard. *How much longer were they going to be in coming to him?* He tried again to remember when he had received his injuries. *Was it daytime? Evening? It must have been night time when he had come round for he seemed to remember laying in moonlight. So like the night of the 'Leasowe Castle' sinking, when the moonlight had been bright as day...* He had seen it, he had lain in it with Toby and Harry and the rest.

The two incidents became confused in his mind and his thoughts began to race making his head hurt, he remembered being afraid that its light was exposing the piles of men who lay awaiting stretchers or burial. *Which night was that? Why had the moonlight gone?*

He was aware of a rustling return and another tread beside. He felt a hand on his shoulder, followed by a man's voice.

'Captain Baird M.O., Gretton. Let's take a look at you shall we?'

He was raised up by strong hands and felt the bandages being unwound from his face, they began to pull, stuck by congealed blood and he heard and felt blunt nosed scissors snipping through them. Light filtered to his eyes but he kept them firmly shut. The bandages covering the wound on his forehead were still in place.

'You can try to open your eyes now,' the doctor said. James hesitated, the urge to free his eyes of wrappings had now left him.

The M.O. rubbed the back of his hand across his face wearily. 'You're not going to do any further damage by opening your eyes trooper,' he said, putting his hand on James' shoulder.

The act of kindness caught James on the raw and to his chagrin he felt tears escaping through his lashes. Dark red channels ran down his cheeks. The M.O's hand tightened on his shoulder. Slowly he forced open his eyelids.

'Well?'

James screwed up his eyes and tried to focus, 'I can see your outline sir, and the nurse, in white, but through a kind of haze.'

'Good chap, the rest will come. Often when the optic nerve gets a bit of a bashing, the sight can be affected, lost even. You're one of the lucky ones.' He examined James eyes with a magnifying glass.

'Well done,' he said. 'Now how does the leg feel?'

'Do I still have it?'

'You bet you do. Had the devil of a job with that, almost took it off, would have been a damn sight easier I can tell you.' He looked up as a tall slim nurse approached. 'With you in a sec sister.'

He turned back to James, 'The leg will take some time, you'll have to be patient, damned if I'll have you ruining some of my best work. Had a French man here helping when you were brought in, a sort of homeopathic doctor, emphatic about not amputating. He treated the wound during my fancy bone setting and stitching, with oils of some kind. Big believer in oils. Same with your head wound, no bone broken there as far as I could make out, fair size gash though. I should say that a smaller lump of shrapnel sliced you as you fell, lucky for you it didn't penetrate, the fall probably saved you.'

He nodded to sister who was hovering. 'Alright sister I'm coming.' He turned his glance back to James, 'Only time will tell whether or not you were fortunate this chap was around. Swore he'd had much success with men and animals alike. Valnet, Dr. Jean Valnet, that's his name. Came well recommended.' He gave the mirthless laugh of the sceptic, then turned and followed sister out of James' vision.

The hospital he learned was housed in a chateau a few kilometres east of St. Emilie. James along with fifty other men lay in orderly rows of beds down each side of a long gallery which was well lit with full length windows. Each day his sight became clearer, much helped, he found, by bathing with diluted drops of the eyebright plant, a treatment left for him by Dr. Valnet.

To James' left was a trooper from his regiment who had been brought in gassed a few days after James was admitted. Between bouts of coughing and retching he was able to tell James of an unsuccessful attack by the Hussars on the 24th September as they had pushed their endeavours towards the Hindenburg Line. The South Notts. had been heavily shelled and gassed during their barrage fire.

He asked James, 'Did you know Harry Brown?'

'Yes, I've gone right through with him. He's not injured is he?'

'Worse than that mate, he just walked into the shell fire.'

'Not Harry?' James felt his body go lifeless with horror.

'They reckon he'd just had a letter from his missus, she's shacked up with some conchie, taken his kids there.'

'O God. He worshiped that woman. We had our first leave together at the end of June. I think things were alright then, he didn't say they weren't.' James put his head in his hands, 'Harry, what a waste.'

One or two surrounding voices commiserated with James.

'You want to thank God you was out of it mate,' the trooper wheezed. 'I know I am, but for what? This evil gas burns your lungs away and what it does to your eyes... Men's and horses' eyes nearly come out of their heads trying to breathe with lungs full of the filth. The lungs can often turn gangrenous.'

From a bed opposite, a man with his leg suspended in a pulley joined in, 'It's wicked what men have been made to suffer in this war, it'll go down in history as massacre on an unprecedented scale.' He lay back on his pillows and stared at the ceiling, 'Horses have had a terrible time too, a lot forget that,' he spoke up with feeling. 'They've done nothing to deserve what they've been made to suffer. There's no animal on earth save perhaps a dog who'll do for man what a horse will do.'

Another voice, 'A bloody dog would get you a long way in this lot mate. I've seen horses up to their shoulders in mud, not a bloody hope in hell of ever getting out, still trying to pull great wagons of timber through shit like that.' The man shook his head, 'I'll never forget the look in a horse's eyes when they have to be dispatched, poor bastards. I'll say they don't deserve it.'

As was usual, others were joining in the conversation. 'A few of us here were at the Somme. An officer told me that 22,000 animals had to be watered at the Somme by the allies.'

'Aye and we had to try and hide them, have you ever tried to hide a horse, a mule or a donkey?'

'War will be with tanks from now on, they can't be beaten. Horses in war are finished.'

'True, the Hussars never made a cavalry charge in this war and never will now.'

'I wouldn't want to see suffering like this again, ever. I've seen horses suffer and by God, I've seen men suffer. I've seen them die together, a tangled mess of bones and guts.'

There was silence for a minute or two, each of the men dwelling on their own horrific memories.

A man a few beds away from James spoke up, 'Tanks are all well and good, but you wouldn't get a tank save a man's life and I heard of a horse that saved a man, injured though it was. The story was told to me when I was in a field hospital near the Somme. It would have been November, 1916. They say that it carried a badly wounded officer away from the battle and walked miles to get him to safety.'

The ward had become silent as the man held their attention. 'It was at the battle of the Ancre, when the allies took Beaumont Hamel, the final end of the battle of the Somme.'

'What became of the horse and the officer?' James asked him.

'That's the strange thing. The officer was eventually taken from a farm where the horse had carried him, into a field hospital and then sent back to England.'

'Well?' the voice from the suspended leg.

'The horse was never recovered by the army. Reckoned they were cagey at the farm, so it was thought the horse had died of its injuries or knowing the frogs, that they'd killed and eaten it anyway.'

'That's the thanks it got is it?'

'They're like carrion here on fallen horses.'

'Poor sods are hungry, that's why.'

'It's all very well to call the French names, but they've had this hell in their country, we haven't, thank God. Think of the civilian deaths, the towns flattened, farmland ruined, the animals and poultry killed and eaten by both sides alike. We've all been glad to get a chicken when we could.'

'And eggs.'

'Anything, to eke out bully beef and biscuits. It's a wonder we haven't all got scurvy.'

'Some of the officers have done a damn sight better, I know that much. Decent billets with no shortages.'

'What it is to be privileged.'

'Talking of the privileged,' a sergeant across the ward, spoke up, 'Did any of you know that rich spectators were allowed to view the battle of the Somme? They rolled up in their expensive vehicles to get a good vantage point. Later they were allowed into operating theatres. Looking for excitement they were heard to say.'

The listeners expressed their disgust.

'My young twin brothers died at the Somme. I heard they screamed for our mother. Is that what the rich bastards enjoyed seeing and hearing?'

'After watching the carnage, 20,000 dead in eight hours, I understand that these people frequented an elegant tea room in a nearby town,' the sergeant said bitterly.

James lay back on his bed, his good leg raised at the knee and stared at the ceiling. He sometimes thought he had heard it all but there was always more. After a while he turned to the narrator of the horse and officer story.

'So that was the end of it then, what you told us?'

'Seems so.' Conversation had resumed in the ward and the storyteller's last words on the subject were barely audible.

'Them that knew about it said this horse was as red as a poppy.'

James felt the blood drain from his face and the skin on the back of his neck contract, 'Was it a stallion?'

'You've heard the story then?'

'I have now. What area did you say it was?'

'A farm, several kilometres from Beaumont Hamel, is what I was told,' he said.

❧ ❧ ❧

The shock of Harry's death and the circumstances which had brought it about had not only grieved James, but would have been an even more serious set back for him were it not for the story of the red stallion, which would not leave him. He was determined to investigate it for himself. Better food and sleep aided his recovery and the wound on his head made good progress, in contrast to his leg which was slow to heal and gave him much pain. His common sense told him that he must exercise the rest of his body, which he did as best he could, encouraging other patients who were able, to do the same. Getting fit had more purpose than ever for him now.

Talk in the ward was usually of the progress of the war. James heard that between the 26th and 27th of September, 217 allied divisions had attacked along the majority of the length of the Western Front, in Flanders, on the Somme, on the Aisle and in the Meuse-Argonne sector where a joint offensive was undertaken by US and French forces. 600,000 of Pressing's troops had been moved from St. Michael to the Argon along with fifteen AEI divisions of 28,000 men per division and 22 French divisions of about 9,000 men per division. 36 German divisions were pinned down, giving the allies a great advantage, including the British attempt to force the Hindenburg Line. The breaking of the first line of the Hindenburg defences, they learned, was down to the efforts of the 46th North Midlands division. This attack, part of a much wider offensive that consisted of five British armies, two French armies, the Belgium army and two US divisions serving with the British Expeditionary Forces culminated on the 4th October with the breaching of the whole line. The British had broken through into open countryside.

The hospital was almost rent apart with cheers. James and other troopers of the South Notts. Hussars were keen to hear of their regiment's advances, whilst at the same time, concerned to learn of the heavy casualties.

By the beginning of November, the bones in James' leg were knitting. The stitches had been removed and almost, James thought, to Doctor Baird's amazement, the leg was now healing well. He was allowed to move about on crutches and spent a large part of his day at one of the windows, watching the motorised ambulances weaving their way through the horse drawn ones on the gravel at the entrance to the chateau.

The name of the man who had related the story of the horse and officer, James learned, was Albert Brown. He also showed a keen interest in the motors.

'After the war's over, I'm going to learn to drive one of them and get me a job in civvy street driving,' he told James.

'Have you ever tried to drive?' James asked him.

'No, but I've watched and now my leg and back are on the mend I'm thinking of trying to get down there and see what I can pick up.'

'Wait for me,' James said. 'There somewhere I want to find before we're moved out of here.'

✄ ✄ ✄

On 11th November, news reached the hospital that the Warwick and South Notts. Yeomanry Machine Gun Battalion had left the village of Baslieu that morning. D and A Companies for Les Fontaines, B Company to join the 199th Brigade at Clairfayts when they were met by the Adjutant, Captain Holden bearing the following message.

'Hostilities will cease at 11.00 hours today, November 11th. Troops will stand fast on line reached at that hour, which will be reported by wire to Headquarters, Fourth Army Advance Guard. Defensive precautions will be maintained. There will be no inter-course of any description with the enemy until receipt of instructions.'

Shortly after 11am when all the church bells in France had rung out, a local farmer brought a horse and cart to the chateau loaded with bottles of wine and gifts from the local inhabitants which they had sacrificed for the patients there. These along with a couple of pigs which the owner of the chateau had rounded up, enabled the momen-tous event to be celebrated on the wards, by the injured, the mutilat-ed, the blind, the gassed and the shell shocked.

Albert was the first to be given the chance to drive. Those who could, attended a thanksgiving service in the gallery which served as James' ward. The few Catholics amongst them had elected to join the locals in a nearby village chapel. Albert offered to drive them there, as the majority of the drivers were attending the service at the chateau. The sergeant in charge allowed Albert a vehicle.

James hoisted himself up into the passenger seat with his crutches. The rest were helped into the back and when the doors had been closed behind them, a slap on the side of the vehicle indicated they could leave.

'This is our chance Jim. This is where it all starts for us mate,' Albert depressed the clutch and put the vehicle into bottom gear. 'The smoother you can release the clutch, the better,' he explained changing up into second. The gravel crunched beneath the tyres and they drove through the gates.

Once clear of the chateau they looked at each other and grinned, 'Yippee!' they shouted in unison.

Their exuberance was infectious and the men in the back began to sing. To a tuneless rendering of *Goodbye Dolly*, the ambulance rocked and swayed over the pitted road towards the village, Albert talking James through every move. Once parked outside the battered chapel of St. Therese, the wounded were unloaded and James struggled down from the cab as the group made their way into the tiny chapel. James sat, his left leg still rigid in splints out in front of him, his head bowed as the familiar words of the Mass began.

'*Introibo ad altare Dei.* I will go unto the altar of God,' and his response, '*Ad Deum, qui laetificat juventutem meam.* To God, who giveth joy to my youth.'

To my youth. His youth, his childhood at the stud with Tom, Annie and Elizabeth. No child could have had a happier childhood. Nor could anyone have experienced a more piercing joy than he, in his passionate love for Beth which had hit him like a thunderbolt. Whatever had happened since could not rob him of those memories. He collected his thoughts as the comforting Latin words continued to fill the church.

'*Spera in Deo, quoniam adhuc confitebor illi: salutare vultus mei, et Deus meus.* Hope in God: for I will still give praise to Him; the salvation of my countenance, and my God.'

He had been spared. He would strive to be young again, strive to push the appalling horrors he had been through to the back of his mind. Get on with his life. But first he needed to accomplish a self imposed mission. He returned his attention to the Mass, joining priest and people in thanksgiving that the heinous conflict had ended.

Despite a week of hard frost following the Armistice, troops on both sides were able to relax, playing football and other recreation, whilst the officers hunted wild boar. James and Albert spent a great deal of their time with the ambulance drivers, eventually managing on occasions to accompany them, ferrying the wounded about. James was a little nearer to his mission.

PART FOUR

AFTERMATH

In November came the Armistice...
Armistice-night hysteria did not touch our
camp much... The news sent me out
walking alone along the dyke above the
marshes of Rhuddlan, cursing and sobbing
and thinking of the dead.

Robert Graves, *Goodbye To All That*

XXIII

Armistice day was many things to many people. Annie and Tom poured over the *Nottingham Evening Post*, Monday, 11th November, reading the headlines in unison.

'*Last shot fired at 11am today. Germany signed the Armistice six hours before time limit expired.*

'*The news for which the world has been so anxiously waiting has come at last, and the war which started so far as Great Britain is concerned, on the night of August 4th, 1914, came to an end this morning with the signing of the armistice by the German emissaries.*

'*The announcement was made by the Premier, the message being received by us at 10.34. Though consisting of not more than twenty words, it conveyed not only the news that the armistice terms had been agreed to, but that the war was to cease on all fronts at the hour which had been fixed upon for the expiration of the time allowed to Germany to make her decision. There had been little doubt as to what Germany's decision would be; all the same Mr. Lloyd George's announcement was received with infinite relief, and universal gratification. The momentous message is as follows:*

'*The Armistice was signed at five o'clock this morning, and hostilities are to cease on all fronts at 11am today.'*

Annie turned to Tom, tears streaming down her face and fell into his arms, he patted her back and made soothing sounds to her whilst his own tears fell into her hair.

'There, there, my love, it's over. They'll be coming home soon now, our boy amongst them, thank God.'

Simultaneously they broke apart and crossed themselves and said the *Te Deum*.

In Lincoln, Elizabeth and her aunt first heard the news by cries in the street outside the house. Aunt Martha pushed open the dining room window and leaned out. A gentleman in a top hat, surrounded by a cheering crowd, called to her, 'The Armistice has been signed ma'am, from eleven o'clock this morning the war will be at an end.'

'Thanks be to God,' Aunt Martha's face broke into a tearful smile as she ran around the table and hugged Elizabeth to her. 'Thanks be to God,' she repeated and hurried into the kitchen to tell cook and the maid.

Elizabeth leaned out of the window, calling thanks to the bearer of the news and laughing along with the crowd around him. She watched in fascination as the little street filled with people, all shouting or singing, many of them waving flags.

On the stroke of eleven, the great bells of Lincoln Cathedral pealed the Steadman Triples, joined by all the church bells in the city, surrounding countryside and throughout the land.

Elizabeth and her aunt stood at the door and listened to the joyful, tumultuous sound, laughing and crying at the same time. In the late afternoon, the bells rang out again and the celebrations went on long into the night and Elizabeth, with no thought of sleep, wrote to Tom and Annie and described the scene.

✂ ✂ ✂

On 13th November, Elizabeth received two letters. The first that she opened was from her friend Florence Smith, dated 11th November, who wrote:

'My dear Elizabeth,

'I hope my letter finds you well at this time of rejoicing and pray that you are being spared the influenza, which has reached epidemic proportions here in Nottingham. At our home, all but mother are down with it. When I say all, that is what I mean Elizabeth dear, my father, my five sisters, my baby brother and me. To save mother from running up two flights of stairs, we are all in one bedroom on the first floor!

'Before breakfast this morning, father read his morning *Nottingham Journal* and told us that the war was to end at 11 o'clock today and although we are still poorly we were so excited as the hour approached. Then the church bells began to ring, the factory buzzers sounded and the newspaper boys were shouting, 'Special! Armistice signed,' and it was all over. We can't imagine what life will be like without a war, can we? And do you know Elizabeth, I'm sure I've mentioned it to you before, we have such a nice family who live opposite to us, Belgians. They came as refugees at the outset of the war, and soon after lunch time, out came a huge Belgian flag fastened to a pole and I shall never forget seeing it through the fog at their bedroom window, its yellow, red and black colours, all creases and folds, it must have been packed away for four years waiting for this wonderful moment. When darkness fell, we could smell the bonfires which had been lit in surrounding areas and could hear people singing *Tipperary* and *Keep the home fires burning.* It seemed that the news has improved the health of all of us and when we settle down for the night we shall know that at last we can sleep peacefully. It has been such an exciting day here Elizabeth, for all we are poorly, and I wanted to share it with you.

'I do hope that James gets home safely. It was such a shock all that time ago, when you told me that he had joined up. What an age it seems since we all learned our Catechism together.

'Write soon. I hope it won't be long before we can visit each other again when normality, (isn't that a wonderful word?) is resumed.

'God bless and keep you safe, much love, Florence.'

'What a lovely letter from dear Florence,' Elizabeth said as she handed it to her aunt to read and cut open the envelope of the second letter. She had already recognised Victoria Burdette's handwriting on the envelope and was still smiling from Florence's letter as she began to read. She felt her vision cloud over the words and the room spin, her hand flew to her heart, 'Oh no, please God, no.'

Aunt Martha looked up, shocked, 'My dear whatever is it?'

Elizabeth slumped back in her chair, head in her hands, tears pouring through her fingers.

'Please, child, what is it?'

Silently Elizabeth passed her the letter. The look of horror which crossed Martha's face as she read Victoria's words was replaced by one of compassion as she went to Elizabeth and put her arm across her shoulders. 'Oh, my dear, it's beyond belief, how utterly tragic and just days before the signing of the Armistice. God help his family.'

❧ ❧ ❧

To Robert the armistice meant the return of supplies to England, but first, having got the task under way, he delegated his minions to continue whilst he took a short spell of leave. He had been dwelling on this for some time, planning in his mind exactly how he would enjoy it and when he docked at Dover it was with purpose that he crossed London from Victoria Station by one of the new mechanised cabs to St. Pancras and then on to Nottingham.

He had already briefed Sybil of his imminent arrival. She greeted him herself and he saw that she was as alluring as ever, her skin taking on a pale translucence, emphasised by the filmy black housecoat she wore.

'Ivan, my dear, how good it is to see you and looking so handsome in uniform.'

He cut her short, 'Did you order my champagne?'

'But of course, it's in the boudoir. You'll have a little something with it, a smoked salmon sandwich perhaps...'

'I've eaten on the train,' he caught hold of her roughly. 'I'll have something with it alright...'

She forced a smile, 'Now don't be impatient, we have hours to ourselves.'

'Ourselves, who said anything about ourselves, I can take on several of you.'

Sybil gave a low giggle, 'You are so very naughty.' She led him up the stairs and into a large room, closing the door behind her. Robert leaned across and turned the key. He glanced around the familiar room which had been the inspiration of much erotic anticipation. In France he had not found anyone who came up to his expectations like Sybil. He observed the closely drawn blinds and gas lamps turned low. The velvet draped couch flanking a marble fireplace in which a fire glowed red. By the couch, a small table bore a few savouries, plates and glasses and three bottles of champagne in an ice bucket. His eyes slid to the large bed which dominated the room, drapes of red and gold silk hung luxuriously from a domed canopy surmounted by red and black ostrich feathers. The sheets and pillows were red satin. The air hung heavily with the musk perfume with which Sybil surrounded herself.

'Here, let me make you more comfortable,' she unbuckled his Sam Brown belt and unbuttoned his jacket, yet before she had completely removed it, he flung himself upon her, kissing her with a violent intensity, his teeth fetching blood to her lips. She extracted herself from him gasping, 'Ivan, behave yourself for a while. Let's have a glass of champagne to celebrate your safe return.'

'Alright, alright, damn it, let's have a drink first, but don't you keep me waiting. I warn you,' his pale eyes glittered dangerously, 'I expect plenty of action from you tonight, my dear Sybil.'

Sybil poured two glasses of champagne and handed one to him before offering a plate of small sandwiches but he rejected them impatiently, downing the contents of the glass in one gulp and urging her to do the same, he continued to refill the glasses and drain them in one swallow until the first bottle was empty.

'There's more,' she said quietly.

He took the glass from her and placed it with his in the fireplace and then in one sweeping move, tore the housecoat from her and threw her onto the bed. She opened her mouth to protest and he pinned her arms above her head with one hand whilst caressing her roughly with the other. Usually, he thought, she would be fighting back like a tiger, hurting him, laughing, challenging him like no other he had known, but tonight she seemed to have no spirit in her. He bent his head and renewed his assault upon her mouth, his teeth grinding upon hers as he ravished her savagely, her cries fuelling his fervour, until he lay across her, spent, and became aware of her sobbing.

'You whining gilt,' he brought his fist down upon her rib cage, his eyes shining, a half smile on his mouth.

'You've gone too far this time, Ivan,' she whimpered.

'You can usually take it, give as good as you get, what the hell's wrong with you?'

'I don't feel quite myself.' She looked up at him and he began to laugh, 'This is a new approach, the simpering Sybil, come on let's see if I can make you really angry, angry enough to try to resist me.' He felt this approach beginning to arouse him again.

She rolled from the bed pulling the tattered robe around her naked body, 'I think not tonight Ivan, I don't feel up to it.'

'Then find me someone who is, damn you, two if you've got them and pass my cigarettes.'

'The only two girls I have who would consider working in pairs are untrained in the ways of this house, I like refined girls here as you know.' She shrugged apparently trying to recover a little of her dignity, 'I've had to employ more girls recently.'

He laughed, 'I bet you have, your reputation precedes you.'

She handed him his cigarettes before staggering to a closet, taking out a fresh robe and wrapping it around herself. She crossed to a dressing table where she touched up her face, wiped the blood from her lip and dragged a comb through her hair, then without looking at him again, left the room

Robert uncorked another bottle of champagne and poured himself a glass, finding the dryness of the wine diluted the taste of Sybil's blood in his mouth. He had almost finished the second bottle when there was a tap on the door. He wrapped a drape from the couch around himself and answered it. Two girls were leaning each side of the door frame. His first impression of them confirmed Sybil's description of their type. They would serve him admirably he thought, as he looked them up and down.

The taller of the two, a stocky redhead stared back at him brazenly. 'Sybil says you are looking for a little rough fun,' she said, giggling at the other girl, a coarse brunette. 'Well, Vi and me can provide that,' she pushed her friend at him before following her into the room and closing the door.

The girls fared little better than Sybil had done, though they gave Robert as good as they got, giggling and fighting across the surface of the red sheets, until Robert finally felt he had realised the hopes he'd had for his leave. He threw a few bank notes onto the bed, the girls fell upon them, their naked buttocks stark against the red sheets as they fought for the money.

A few minutes later, Robert paused by the front door and checked his appearance in the hall mirror. He made a few adjustments to his dress and then pushed an envelope behind the mirror for Sybil as was his usual custom. Picking up his case, he opened the door to leave, admitting an elderly man carrying a black leather bag.

XXIV

Jacques Vautrin looked across the kitchen table at his wife. He poured himself a cognac. 'I don't like it Monique. We were sworn to secrecy two years ago, not only giving our word, but accepting money.' He drained the glass, refilled it to the brim and stared into it. 'I only ever used the money for the horse,' he said at length, 'Whatever foodstuff could get my hands on for him and then there was the cost of bringing Henri's closed wagon and team of work horses all the way over here so we could move the horse without him being seen.'

'It's seven months now since we heard from *le capitan*, he has not been out of touch with us for so long.'

'What are we to do if he's been killed?'

She had put into words Jacque's fears and for a while they sat without speaking, the silence broken only by the crackle of logs in the hearth.

Monique put her head in her hands, 'What do you think will happen to us if we are found out? If the English *capitan* is dead, we shall have no one to speak for us.'

'Whether the English *capitan* is dead or alive we'll have no one to speak for us. He would be in as much trouble as we are, we've done wrong and we knew we were doing wrong all along. The horse is still army property.'

'What should we have done?' she asked him.

'Probably what we told the sergeant who came to investigate, that the horse had died of its injuries, and implied we had eaten it. I go cold when I remember the horse was in one of our sheds, sick, when he called. I couldn't bring myself to tell him, I know he would have shot it. We could have saved ourselves so much trouble if we'd let him, or killed it as you suggested at the time. Remember?'

'I didn't know the horse then, nor did I realise the full significance of what it had done. Oh, I'm not excusing myself and God knows the meat would have been welcome, no one could have blamed us, eating a horse as badly injured as that.'

Jacques offered her the bottle, she pushed it away impatiently, 'No, and you've had enough, drinking too much isn't going to help us now, is it?'

He shook his head, 'Now that trooper has been here, he'll come again. His friend told me in his attempt at French, that they have covered a complete circle in this region in their efforts to track down the farm where the horse came to.'

'What's his interest? Do you think he's a reporter or something?'

'I wouldn't think so, though I have a gut feeling that we are soon to find out. Whatever it is, it must be important to him, tracking us down whilst he's not yet recovered from his injuries.' Jacques toyed with his glass, 'Weird, and yet there's something about that trooper which reminded me of myself.'

Monique managed a faint smile, 'Oh Jacques, how you flatter yourself, much as I love you, never have you had the looks of that boy. In all my life, I've not seen such eyes, even on a girl, so honest, so grey and the lashes...'

'Stop talking rubbish woman, you're getting carried away now. I didn't mean in looks, but no matter, we've got enough to worry about without you fantasising. *Mon Dieu*, he could be our undoing, never mind his eyes.'

'Don't say that, it makes my stomach churn.' She bit her lip and looked hard at him, 'I think I will have a cognac after all.'

✄ ✄ ✄

Elizabeth found the letter she was endeavouring to write to Mr. and Mrs. Brown the hardest of her life. Since receiving the terrible news of Saxon's death, she had scarcely stopped crying for her beloved friend. The waste paper basket by the *bonheur du jour* in her bedroom was full of screwed up attempts, eventually she settled for one and asked her aunt's opinion.

'I think so darling, please God it will comfort them to know that Saxon's friends are grieving for him too. Also, that you are planning to visit them after their period of family mourning.'

Elizabeth nodded dumbly and commenced writing a short letter to Victoria which she intended to take to the post along with her letter for the Browns. It came as quite a surprise the next morning to receive another letter from Victoria. Elizabeth felt her heart lurch as she recognised the writing on the envelope.

'Will you open it for me, aunt?' she asked, passing the envelope to Martha.

'Oh dear,' Martha said, as she commenced reading.

'What now, please, not more.' Elizabeth paced the room, wringing her hands.

'Do sit down dear,' Aunt Martha advised her.

'Tell me.'

'It's Captain Oakley.'

'Is he dead?'

Aunt Martha evidently mistook the inflexion in Elizabeth's voice for distress.

'No, no, he isn't dear. It seems that he came over for a short leave and has caught the influenza. Victoria writes, 'Poor Mrs. Oakley is at her wits end and has engaged a nurse solely to look after Robert as they dare not expose the squire to the epidemic.'' She handed the letter to Elizabeth. 'Would you believe it Elizabeth, all the way back from France for this. You would wonder wherever he could have picked it up.'

⚜ ⚜ ⚜

Some days after his initial visit, James was attempting to talk Albert into returning with him to the farmhouse.

'It was to this farm that the stallion took the officer, that much we do know.' James lay on his bed and stared at the ceiling. The splints had been removed from his leg and mobility was gradually returning, though it still gave him a great deal of pain.

'Listen, mate, when we can get a vehicle, I'd sooner go into the nearest town and find us a couple of girls, even visit one of the houses of hospitality,' Albert said, looking at James covertly.

The trooper to James' left laughed dryly, 'You want to keep away from those places sonny, there's more swaddys with the clap than there's been fatalities in this bloody war.'

'Mind your own sodding business,' Albert glared at him, 'Anyway what's a dose of the clap.'

'If it's syphilis, you'd soon find out what. Listen to me and don't risk it.' He finished his advice with a searing bout of coughing.

Albert slapped his back a couple of times and turned to James, 'What I mean Jim is, it's such a shame when we get the chance of a drive, to waste it on some bloody incident that happened two years ago. I can't understand why you're so interested. I almost wish I'd never told you, it's all you think about these days.'

'You're right. Has it occurred to you that I have my reasons?'

'I can't think for the life of me what they'd be,' Albert grumbled as he rolled a thin cigarette. He didn't look up from his task until he had licked the paper, stuck it down and lit it, then poked at the depleted contents of his tobacco tin.

'I'll give you my tobacco ration, I'm stopping smoking so you're welcome to it,' James offered.

Albert re-examined the contents of the tin before replacing the lid, 'Tell you what I'll do,' he said, 'I'll get round the sergeant to let you have a motor today and I'll do him some driving work tomorrow. I might just pull in a visit to the town.' He carefully removed the ash from his cigarette, 'I only hope your leg is up to it.'

'I'll be fine,' James told him. 'We might not have much longer here, I can't afford to miss this chance. They could move us out anytime, bound to. I think they've only left us this long because there are so many wounded to move out.'

Albert held the stub of the cigarette in his finger nails, drew on it and dropped it onto James' bed, 'Bloody hell, that's hot.' He batted the bedding.

'They'll move us all out for sure if you set the place on fire,' James thumped out the sparks, then resumed the conversation. 'It's just that I want to hear a bit more about it, the end of the story if you like.'

'We know the end, they ate it, they told us so.'

❧ ❧ ❧

James found the drive hard on his leg, which he found had not healed enough to work the clutch and brake without considerable pain. He had become used to Albert sitting close and working these foot controls for him with his own good right leg. His body became bathed in sweat as he gripped the steering wheel whilst the vehicle jolted over the tracks.

As soon as he pulled into the yard, James sensed they had been expecting him to return. Monique moved a lace curtain aside and watched him make his ungainly descent from the ambulance.

Jacques walked purposefully across the yard pushing a wheelbarrow full of muck with a fork stuck into it. He barely acknowledged James, making it clear, James thought, that he had no intention of being cajoled into talking, or leaving his yard work.

'Good afternoon *m'sieur*,' James began cheerfully.

Jacques merely grunted, his pace didn't alter as he pushed the barrow past him.

James limped alongside, '*M'sieur*, you'll have a drink with me?'

The man had a moderate understanding of English, but the bottle of cognac in James' hand bore a French label, which he understood perfectly.

He slowed to a stop and rested the barrow on its back legs, 'There's nothing I can tell you, that I have not already done. The horse was mortally wounded. It died of its injuries and we ate it, we had no food. Whether you, English, like it or not, that's what happened.'

James' knowledge of French was limited, having only recently arrived in the country, although he had made a considerable effort during the time he had been confined to bed at the chateau.

'I wouldn't blame you *m'sieur*, times have been hard. Just have a drink with me and tell me about that day. I promise you I have good reason to ask.' James shrugged in a helpless gesture, guaranteed to appeal to the Frenchman and then turned towards the window and smiled at Monique as he held up the bottle. 'Please *m'sieur*, drink with me - to peace.'

The man sighed and turned towards the house, washed his hands at a stone sink outside the door then scraped off his boots on the step and gestured for James to follow him in. Monique inclined her head towards James, beckoning him to sit beside her on a horsehair couch by the fire and pointed to a scrubbed kitchen chair for Jacques. James offered the bottle to her and she accepted it graciously and set three small glasses on the table.

After they had toasted each other, James leaned towards Jacques, 'About the horse. You say he died? All I ask is that you tell me a little more of the story.'

'There is no more to tell,' Jacques drained his glass and poured himself another. 'The horse was practically finished when it came here, by the time we had made provision for *le capitan*, it had collapsed in the yard. We could not rouse it. By the morning it was dead, lying in the yard out there, soaked and swollen with the rain.'

'What colour was it?

Jacques was on his third glass, 'Colour, English? When it was wet it looked very dark, but dry...' his lined face broke into a smile, 'Dry, it became the colour of the red maple.'

James' heart seemed to miss a beat. 'It had no markings, just as red as a horse could be?'

The man stared into his glass and slowly began to nod, raising his eyes to James, 'Yes, and what breeding.'

Monique glared at him and then at James, 'Ignore the old fool, English. A glass or two of cognac and he makes no sense.'

James said quietly, 'And when you talk low to the horse, he listens, he takes no tit bit unless maybe you leave it in the manger and when he hears your tread, he whinnies twice.'

Jacques stared at him, 'How do you know these things?'

'Because I was at his birth, I helped to break him in, I schooled him, trained him, formed a relationship with him and just as he was coming into his own, someone sold us out, betrayed us. I saw him commandeered, too young by far, way out of turn, breaking the hearts of those who were connected with him.'

Jacques looked hard into James' eyes. If not all of the words meant anything to him, James' sincerity did, 'What did you call the horse of which you speak?'

'His name is Ri Rua, he's from old Irish bloodlines, it means Red King.'

'Jacques eyes were moist, '*Le Rouge.*'

James leaned forward, 'Please *m'sieur* tell me about him.'

Jacques sighed and avoided Monique's eye, 'It took many months for the horse to heal, he almost died, I prayed over that animal, I besought God to let it live for what it had done. May God forgive me but I prayed harder for the horse than I did for *le capitan*. I left him to Monique and as I did right by the horse, so she did by the man.' He took a swallow of cognac, 'By the time the burnt arrows had grown out of its hooves I'd taken him over to my wife's cousin, Henri, where the good spring grass and clean air and quiet did much to restore him.' He sat quietly for a moment and then said simply, 'We have a saying in these parts, '*Pour que la Terre garde son empreinte...* it is the right of every animal to touch the earth.''

James nodded, acknowledging his wisdom, before asking. 'Who else knows that the horse survived?'

Jacques drew a deep breath, 'Only *le capitan* and Bridges... his soldier servant?'

'Yes.'

'*Le capitan* sent the soldier servant with money, hoping that the horse was still alive. He saw we cared for him, hadn't given him up as we might have done. He told us that *le capitan* was to be sent back to England to a hospital and that he would continue to bring money from him.'

James whistled through his teeth, 'What does he intend doing with the horse now that the war is over?'

Jacques looked at him in amazement, 'Why, take him to England of course, *le capitan* owes his life to the horse.' He stared at the window which overlooked the yard, the tears which had threatened earlier now spilled into the stubble on his cheeks, '*Mon Dieu*, what a horse. He barely made it into this yard, he was so close to death having sustained a terrible wound and lost much blood, yet he had carried a mortally wounded man with more compassion than many men would have done, away from the shell fire, away from the battle, to the safety of this place.'

Jacques spread his hands, 'What could I do, other than my best for him? He is an exceptional animal and I know horses as did my *grandpère* who raised me. It's not just his breeding and presence that captured me, but his temperament and to the horse's eternal credit, *le capitan* lived.'

Monique leaned towards James, 'We've heard nothing from him for almost seven months, occasionally it's been a few weeks, but never this long.' Her voice faltered, 'We fear he must have been killed.'

Her words hung between them. The ticking of the wall clock seemed to James to dominate the room, gradually, sounds from outside began to challenge it, the rattle of a cow chain, the grunt of a pig, a cockerel crowing in the distance.

'I must see the horse,' James said eventually.

'But *le capitan*?'

'Have you made any enquiries about him?'

Monique took James' face in her hands and stared into his eyes, 'No. No enquiries. That would be breaking trust, a trust we have honoured for two years. How can we do that, English?'

'My name madame, is Gretton, James Gretton.'

'How James, can we do this?'

'I understand madame and agree with you. All I ask is to see the horse. I give you my word that I mean no harm to you, or to anyone involved.'

She took her hands from his face and looked to Jacques as James asked, 'Where is he?'

After what seemed an age, Jacques told him, 'Near Sombrin.'

✣ ✣ ✣

Elizabeth burst into the sitting room where her aunt was dozing in front of the fire. She tore off her coat as she rushed her words. 'Aunt Martha, there are to be auctions around the country of horses being returned from the war, surplus to army requirements.'

Martha raised herself upright in the chair and stared at Elizabeth. 'How do you know?'

'Because many of our patients have local newspapers sent to them from different parts of the country. We often borrow them to read at break times. It seems the sales are going to be sporadic and so I must keep looking out for them. There's a sale in Nottingham next week and one in Leicester the following week. I intend to go to both of them and any others I can get to know of.'

It was apparent that Martha did not share the fervour which the news had aroused in her niece. 'Darling, be realistic. It wouldn't be right for an unaccompanied young woman to be going around auction sales. Your dear Mama wouldn't have entertained it.' Martha raised her hand to silence Elizabeth as she continued, 'The chances, my dear, of any of your horses being returned to this country are, I should say, practically nil. Please listen to me.'

Elizabeth set her jaw. It was the first time, she and her aunt had differed, but she felt determined to have her way over this issue.

'Please Aunt, bear with me. It's my only chance to try to find any of our horses which may have been spared. So very many have been killed and maimed. I understand that they are only bringing the best of them back, the remainder are to be slaughtered,' her voice faltered, 'that's how they are to be repaid. I wonder if any of ours are amongst those?' She put her head in her hands, 'O God, we shall never know.' She looked at her aunt, 'So many horses - what have they done to deserve any of it? I read only last week that this war has just about wiped out Welsh Cobs. Can you imagine what that means, an entire native breed practically gone forever?' Elizabeth lowered her voice, 'They took a Welsh Cob from us.'

'I know they did my dear, that day must have been terrible for you.' She looked at Elizabeth kindly, 'I fear that you are going to open up a lot of old wounds if you try to pursue what I really believe will be a hopeless cause.'

'You may be right Aunt, but I have to do it. I owe them that. Please try to understand. I wouldn't hurt you for the world but,' she repeated, 'please try to understand.'

The day ended without agreement. As she lay in bed that night, Elizabeth knew that although she appreciated her aunt's dilemma, a restlessness was building up inside her, along with the obsession to search for some of what she had lost and begin to think about plans to rebuild on what she had left. Four years of war had not diminished the void left by the horses which had been so unfairly commandeered, neither had those years lessened her detestation of Robert Oakley, who she now fully believed to have been responsible. She could think of no reason that could have provoked such malice from him, or, she thought with a shudder, such unspeakable violence. James had tried to warn her, he had seen in Robert what she had not. Her new found hope, combined with such conflicting emotions kept her awake into the small hours.

The situation reached a compromise. Elizabeth wrote to Tom and Bob and asked if they would attend surplus army horse auctions in the Nottinghamshire and Derbyshire areas. Back up arrangements were made for Mr. Neeson's office to forward a float for any purchase and to cover expenses. Any horse or horses bought to be taken by rail to Gatthorpe. With Martha's reluctant agreement Elizabeth was to travel to auctions further afield, accompanied by Wilfred.

The first sale she attended was at Leicester Horse Repository. It did not take Elizabeth long to discover that none of the surplus army horses were known to her, though she did feel, to the credit of the army that the animals were well fed and cared for, but many of them rolled their eyes and showed signs of stress. Sales attended by Tom and Bob at Nottingham and Derby drew blanks. Birmingham, Coventry, Sheffield and Manchester sales, covered by Elizabeth and Wilfred also proved fruitless. Returning by rail from the latter, Elizabeth slumped into a seat in the corner of the carriage felt unbelievable disappointment and defeat.

'I'm beginning to think that Aunt Martha was right,' she said wearily. 'I'm not going to find any of my horses am I Wilfred?'

Wilfred smiled encouragingly, 'Don't give up Elizabeth, stranger things have happened. Maybe the next sale. Where is it to be held?'

'We have to wait for them appearing in the press or *Horse and Hound*. I don't think they are intended to be ongoing.'

A waiter came down the corridor calling passengers for dinner. Elizabeth unfastened her bag and took out their sandwiches.

'Come on,' Wilfred said, standing up, 'I'll treat you to dinner, cheer us up eh?'

✄ ✄ ✄

The move which James predicted came more swiftly than he and Albert had anticipated. News that the gravely ill and injured at the chateau were to be taken to hospitals in England and the walking wounded sent home on leave which would probably be extended until demobilisation was received by James with dismay and Albert with elation.

'I must have a vehicle,' James said, 'Just once more.'

'You've got a girl on haven't you?' Albert accused him. 'I'll bet she's connected with that farm, you sly devil, there's been more to this than you've let on, hasn't there?'

'Never mind all that,' James said impatiently, 'Be a mate and help me this last time.'

Albert was sorting through his meagre possessions, 'What are you offering?'

'I've nothing left to barter, come on Albert, you can get round that sergeant a hell of a lot better than I can. He still thinks my leg isn't up to it no matter how much I offer to help out with trips.'

'Where will you be going?' Albert asked craftily.

'Well, in the direction of the farm.'

'I knew it, you cunning old bugger.'

It was a few anxious days before James got his opportunity, during which he had been expecting orders to move out at any time. Making sure the motor's tank was filled with petrol, he left the chateau early, before anyone could interfere with his plans.

Jacques and Monique were having breakfast when he arrived at the farmhouse.

'*Mon Dieu*, I doubt I can spare time to take you over to Henri's today my friend, and how can I let him know at such short notice?' Jacques dunked bread into a bowl of coffee, 'Couldn't you have got word to us that you were coming?'

'No, I couldn't unfortunately,' James told him. 'It's a devil of a job to get a motor and we've had news that we're being sent home at any time.'

Jacques sucked in his breath and looked at Monique. She knew him well enough to interpret his look. 'Alright, Jacques, I'll do the pressing jobs, see to the stock and the likes. Take James to see the horse, the boy will never rest if he has to go home with this unresolved.'

To James, the journey seemed interminable, for the going was slow due to icy roads. Whilst he was frantically anxious to see the horse, use of the clutch and brake pedals still gave him serious pain, causing him to clench his teeth and dash the sweat from his face impatiently. Although it was now December and the countryside looked stark, he was fascinated by the unspoilt landscape, his main impression of France so far being the desecrated and war torn sites of battle. The further they travelled, the more this was apparent. By midday they arrived at a tidy holding with well tended fields fenced off with post and rails. James scanned the place expectantly. Cows grazed to the left of the drive and on the horizon James could see what looked like a few mares and foals by a large brick and timber barn.

Following Jacques' directions he drove into a yard, with buildings on two sides and a timber framed farmhouse on the other. Whilst he was still struggling out of the vehicle, Jacques had made his way to the farmhouse and was calling Monique's cousin.

Henri appeared at the door evidently in the middle of his lunch for he had a large checked napkin tucked down his neck. After much cheek kissing and back slapping, Jacques beckoned James over and made the introductions. Henri pumped James' hand up and down, before steering him into the house. James ducked under the low door and found he had to stoop in the heavily beamed kitchen.

A motherly figure in an overall got up from the table and insisted James take her place and before the men had finished introducing him to her, she had set a bowl of broth in front of him with a chunk of crusty bread.

'A glass of wine, English?'

'James Gretton, madame.'

'A glass of wine, James?' she enquired again and without waiting for a reply filled a glass from a barrel and handed it to him. Jacques was receiving the same hospitality at the other side of the table. Lunch over, Henri asked if James would like to see around the farm.

'I would *m'sieur*, especially the horses.'

James found the place a credit to Henri and his family, comparing it with his memories of the O'Malley yards. It was, however, the horses that excited his interest. In and around the barn were three mares, all with young foals of exceptional quality.

James complimented Henri and asked, 'The stallion *m'sieur*, the sire of these youngsters, I would like to see him.'

Henri looked from one to the other and then whispered hoarsely to Jacques, 'I wrote to you, Jacques, two days ago and enclosed a letter from *le capitan*. You've obviously not received the letters yet. The stallion has gone. *Le capitan* sent his soldier servant Bridges and a civilian groom for him. I understood that arrangements had been made for him to travel to England.'

James lowered himself onto a bench by the wall of the barn. Was this where it was all to end, his hopes of tracing Rua, if indeed the stallion was Rua. Now he would never know. He looked to Henri, 'Where have they taken him to in England, *m'sieur*?'

Henri's face clouded, he turned to Jacques and began speaking to him in rapid French. James watched them, knowing he had little hope this time of picking up anything they were saying.

Eventually, Jacques sat down beside James, 'I've had great difficulty persuading my cousin-in-law that you are trustworthy. He is naturally very concerned about an outsider knowing our business.' He spread his hands, 'We have done wrong whilst doing right.'

The logic of his words was not lost on James.

'I have told him of your connection with a horse of the description of *le Rouge*. He is a horseman, he understands.' Jacques looked to Henri who nodded. He turned to James, 'They have taken the horse to Hertfordshire, to *le Capitan* Thorpe.'

'I shall need a letter,' James said.

XXV

Aunt Martha and Wilfred dropped Elizabeth at the bottom of Oakley village.

'You're sure darling that you want to go alone?' her aunt asked anxiously.

'Quite sure,' Elizabeth leaned forwards and kissed her cheek, then squeezed Wilfred's arm, 'Thank you for bringing me.'

Wilfred smiled at her indulgently, 'Always a pleasure, Elizabeth.'

'So we'll pick you up from Tom and Annie's around four, although I do think you should have let Annie know that you intended to call,' Aunt Martha remonstrated.

'Annie always makes me welcome,' Elizabeth assured her, 'and they don't go far.'

Aunt Martha adjusted her scarf, 'If you're sure... my but it's cold, thank goodness you listened to me and wrapped up warmly.'

Elizabeth watched them drive away, raising a hand to the retreating car whilst dread at the prospect of seeing Saxon's family overwhelmed her. She set off through the village where so many of her memories were rooted. There was no-one about and she walked briskly, when she passed the stud, she did not falter, but continued past, knowing that she would be calling when her mission was over. Her thoughts instead, turned to the Browns. She felt tears gathering and dashed them away impatiently, determined to control her grief in consideration of the family of her beloved friend. Walking up the drive to the farm, whilst still some distance from the farmhouse and buildings, Elizabeth sensed a forlorness about the place. The trees which lined the drive looked gaunt, beyond them the surrounding fields were bare, as though they too were in mourning.

❧ ❧ ❧

Later, when walking back down the drive, her face was wet with tears. She had found that she could not hold them back at the Browns and she and Mrs. Brown had clung together and wept.

Elizabeth had one more appointment to keep before seeing Tom and Annie. She turned into Earth Lane, wrapping her coat around her and pulling on her hood. The day was almost as cold as the day when Saxon and herself had taken their last walk together. Feeling wretched and empty, Elizabeth made her way beneath the giant beeches to the fallen tree by the side of the bridle path where they had sat and talked and vowed to meet when the war was over. She sat in the same place and closed her eyes, seeing again his dear familiar face as it had been that day, his blue eyes filled with concern for her. She felt his presence so close that she could almost hear his voice and his laughter, feel his sincerity and his wonderful bumbling kindness. She dropped her head into her hands and sobbed unrestrainedly, cruelly aware of his absence by her side. The needless, wicked waste of his life and the lives of so many young men like him, tore at her.

She remained at the site of the rendezvous until she was stiff with cold, retreating into her grief and determination to honour the promise she had made to her friend. Suddenly, she was shocked from her inertia, sensing an approaching presence. She opened her eyes and couldn't believe what she saw, for Major and Dolcis, her father's dogs bounded up to her. Instinctively, she looked around, expecting to see Tom taking them on their favourite run, but she could see no-one on the bridlepath. She took off her gloves and ran her fingers over their ears whilst she talked to them. Then looking up again, she saw a figure silhouetted against the pale sky, on top of the bank, behind the trees. It was not Tom. It was James.

Even from the distance she knew instinctively that he was as shocked to see her as she was to see him. He had stopped in his tracks and for a moment she thought he was going to turn and go back the way he had come. She stood up, her legs weak and trembling. Her breathing became shallow and she felt as though her heart would burst. He was in uniform, closed neck khaki tunic, breeches and greatcoat. Elizabeth couldn't take her eyes from him, how he had matured, how confident his stance. Her long cherished feelings for him surged through her and she strove to caution herself, fearful of his rejection.

He half turned, whistling the dogs. She couldn't see him go like that, she tried to move towards the bank but her legs felt leaden.

'James,' her voice was hoarse with crying and barely audible.

He must have heard her, she realised, for he turned and she felt he almost shrugged as he began his descent of the bank. It was then that she saw his terrible limp, emphasised by the steep incline and her heart went out to him. She turned her attention to the dogs who had bounded back to her, lest she embarrass him. He was now walking towards her, his limp less pronounced on the level ground.

'Oh, God help me,' she thought, 'I've waited for more than four years for this. My darling James.'

He stood before her and for a fleeting moment it was as though the past four years didn't exist, hadn't existed, then the moment passed and she was grievously aware that those years did exist and had come between them, with all that she didn't understand. She raised her eyes to his, she had often felt that his grey eyes couldn't have had the intensity with which she remembered them, but now, as their eyes met, she was struck by their intensity and knew that her memory had not failed her. Once more she felt the long forgotten twist in her stomach of great love for him. Her eyes moved to the livid scar on the left side of his forehead and compassion overwhelmed her, she lifted her hand to reach out to him, but he drew back from her.

'Annie said you'd been injured.'

'It's nothing,' his tone was sharp.

'James?'

'Miss Elizabeth.' It was as though he had plunged a knife into her, she gasped at the hurt he had inflicted with his words. She sank down onto the log.

'Please James, don't.'

He looked away, through the winter branches, the hall could be seen on the rise of the next hill.

'Been to see the invalid son and heir, I would guess, by your tears.' There was cynicism in his voice which she had never heard from him.

She bit her lip and twisted a handkerchief in her hands, 'No. I've been to see Saxon's family.'

'I was sorry about Saxon.'

'I promised him, I would meet him here when the war was over. I kept my promise.'

He was quiet for a while before asking, 'You keep some promises then?'

She looked up at him, 'What do you mean?'

He laughed wryly, 'I think you know well enough, Miss Elizabeth.'

'Why do you call me that, James?' Elizabeth felt bewildered, out of her depth, what an awful way to meet, he was so bitter against her. How he must hate her. Why, why, why? She began to cry again and turned away from him lest he should see.

'I must go, I've some packing to do, that's why I brought the dogs early.'

'I had planned to call and see Tom and Annie,' she said miserably.

'They'll be pleased to see you,' he said, turning and calling up the dogs. They walked in silence back along Earth Lane and down the village towards the stud. Elizabeth felt as though she was walking in a dream, James by her side, but not the James she knew. Gone was the boy who had loved her with both gentleness and strength and a commitment she had believed equalled her own. Even his appearance had changed, how much taller he had grown than her, how broad his shoulders had become. She was acutely aware of his presence, of his absolute masculinity which had first awakened her emotions when she had been just sixteen.

She glanced at him under her eyelids, his face was wet with sweat and she knew he was in agony, yet she almost had to run to keep up with him, he was striding out so purposefully. His limp grieved her and she covered her mouth with her hand, lest she call out to stop causing himself such pain.

She knew that he couldn't wait to be away from her, to get her to his family and then disappear. What could have happened between them to cause such pitiless hostility? Firmly, she reminded herself of her promise to God, that if he were spared, she would never, all her life, be unforgiving towards him. She wondered if he was in love again, had met a girl he would look at as he had once looked at her, make love to as he had made love to her. A girl who would return his love, his caresses, yet whom she knew, could not love him more than she had done, and, she thought in anguish, still did.

He opened the heavy gates for her and then went off to take the dogs back to their kennels. Elizabeth made her way through the top yard and round to the cottage. The door was ajar and she could hear voices from the inside. She called and Annie appeared.

'Elizabeth, what a lovely surprise, come along in.'

'You're busy...' Elizabeth indicated to a few boxes and packages piled up inside the doorway.

'They're James's. He's home Elizabeth, thanks be to God.' Annie took her arm and led her inside. 'Here I am in the middle of writing a letter to you.'

'I'd just written to you Annie, I didn't see the point of posting it when I was seeing you and there's so much I want to talk to you about.' Elizabeth felt in her bag and handed a letter to Annie. Annie slipped it into the pocket of her skirt.

James had not returned, but Tom crossed the room to clasp her hand, 'This is a surprise,' he said, smiling at her. 'James is home, on sick leave, it seems to be taking a long time for demobilisation.'

She nodded, 'I've already seen him, he was in Earth Lane with the dogs. I've been to call on Saxon's family.'

'Oh Elizabeth, how are they now?'

'Grief stricken Annie, isn't it terrible?'

Annie's face crumpled, 'We went to see them last week, how can you comfort a family who have suffered such a loss?'

Tom sighed, 'They will appreciate your visit Elizabeth. Richard Brown said that they have received some consolation from the support they've had from so many who knew Saxon. He was well liked, one of the best.'

They were quiet for a while as the awful cost of war weighed upon them.

'One of the very best,' Elizabeth agreed, fighting back tears, 'I wrote that I would call this week, but as it happened, today I got the chance of a lift with Aunt Martha's brother-in-law, Wilfred, he was coming over to Nottingham in his motor car. Aunt Martha is with him, they're going to pick me up here if that's alright?'

'Alright? Of course it is. Come and sit down my dear, we're about to take a break, it will be just like the old days,' Annie said.

But it wasn't like those days, Elizabeth thought sadly. She was on edge expecting James to appear at any moment and whilst half of her longed to see him again, the other half recoiled from the coldness she knew she could expect from him.

'You say James is packing? Is he moving?'

Annie looked to Tom, who answered, 'He's got a place, across the river at Wilford.'

Elizabeth nodded dumbly as Annie spoke again, 'He has his reasons Elizabeth...' She was interrupted by James' return. He strode into the kitchen, evidently catching the last of Annie's sentence.

'Ma,' he looked at Annie sharply and acknowledged Elizabeth with a nod.

Tom and Annie looked at James in bewilderment and then at each other, their eyes pained and uncomprehending. James took off his greatcoat and hung it on the door, then mumbled an excuse and went upstairs. Elizabeth could hear boxes being dragged across the floors. He didn't reappear, although Annie called up to him that they had made tea.

✄ ✄ ✄

James surveyed his bedroom, the room where he had, in the past, thought of and dreamt of Elizabeth and of the intensity of his love for her. He thought of the fateful night he had spent in the room after receiving her last message to him, delivered with such fiendish pleasure by Robert Oakley. Now she was in the room below, no more than a stranger. He sat on the bed and closed his eyes. He saw her in many situations. The night of the ball when she had looked like a dream, riding the red stallion as if she were part of it, lying in the hayfield looking up at him, in his arms in the loft, his lips upon hers. He gave an anguished sigh and put his head in his hands. Still the thoughts invaded his mind. Seeing her some months ago at the railway station, he couldn't have imagined that she had become even more beautiful and then today when he had crested the bank and looked down at her in Earth Lane and later faced her, seeing her lovely face wet with tears.

'Why had he been so hateful?'

'For what she had done to him of course.'

Yet, despite her callous rejection and all he had done to shut her out of his mind through the years of war, the memories of her, he knew, had sustained him. Please God, may he never see her again, enabling him to get on with his life. He must say goodbye to her with as good a grace as he could. He began to sort his belongings in a frenzy, forcing further thought from his mind.

Feeling uncomfortable in the cottage for the first time in her life, Elizabeth rose when she had finished her tea. 'I must see Mrs. Bailey,' she glanced at the longcase clock by the hearth, 'I shall just about have time before Aunt Martha and Wilford arrive. Please excuse me, Annie, Tom.'

As soon as Elizabeth had left, Tom strode to the stairs door, 'James, will you come down here please?'

Annie, hearing James' feet on the stairs, shook her head ruefully.

Tom challenged him, 'Just what do you think you're doing James? How could you be so churlish to Elizabeth, my God, you've grown up with her, whatever has got into you?'

'Leave it Pa,' James pulled off his tunic in the warm kitchen and opened the neck of his shirt.

Annie began to cry. 'Please Ma, leave it.'

He had scarcely spoken when there was a tap at the door. Annie opened it to Elizabeth.

'Mrs. Bailey isn't there,' she said.

Annie clamped a hand around her forehead, 'I'm sorry Elizabeth, I quite forgot that she was going over to see Jenna today.'

Elizabeth was not listening. Her eyes were fixed on the medallion around James' neck. Her jaw dropped and she looked absolutely incredulous.

'They have kept in touch right through the war...' Annie's voice trailed off as she became aware of the atmosphere.

The silence which followed was broken by Elizabeth. 'Where did you get the medallion of St. James that you gave to me?'

James looked across the room at her, his eyes frigid, 'From Robert Oakley of course, the day you gave it to him to throw into my face.'

Elizabeth's voice became strained and high, 'You say that I gave it to him. The last time I saw the medallion was the day when the squire collapsed, the same day that Robert Oakley attacked me and tore it from my neck and struck me with such violence that I was only half conscious.' Instinctively she put her hand to the side of her face.

James stared at her, 'You stayed at his home after he did that?' His question was an accusation.

'I had a fever, because I'd wandered for hours, dazed. He left for France, if he hadn't I would have crawled home somehow, whatever Doctor Morley had said.'

'But you became reconciled with him?' His voice was low.

'I did not. I haven't laid eyes on him from that day and I never shall. I loathe him. He might have taken my home, but not me, never me.'

'I'll kill him,' James grabbed his tunic and reached for a twelve bore from the gun rack, pocketed a handful of cartridges and was out of the house before any of them could prevent him.

Tom pulled his coat from the back of the door, 'My God,' he said, 'We've got to stop him.' He dashed through the door calling after James. Annie looked at Elizabeth, 'Whatever is this all about?' Elizabeth laid her hand on Annie's arm and then followed Tom.

James reached the hall only seconds before them. One of the gardeners was pushing a large wheelbarrow full of tools round the gravel towards the outbuildings. He recognised James in the failing light.

'James, good to see you home. Terrible news isn't it?'

James frowned as he rushed by. The gardener's next words brought him to a halt, 'The young captain has just died of the 'flu.'

XXVI

Later, after Elizabeth had left, Tom, Annie and James were seated around the range.

'I think James, the time has come for some explanations. Just what had happened when you left for the army?'

James sat for a while and stared into the fire, he felt totally deflated, filled with self loathing. He looked at his hands and then clenched them and dropped his head onto them.

They sat in silence for a while and then in a broken voice, he began to tell them. He told them of the great love he had felt for Elizabeth and which he had believed was totally reciprocated, of his humiliation at the hands of Robert Oakley, of his devastation at Elizabeth's disloyalty and the cruel rejection by which she had spurned him. He told them of his feeling of total worthlessness at their hands and of his decision to leave at once.

'But she did none of this,' Tom said quietly.

The silence was disturbed only by Annie's quiet sobbing.

'I know that now. God help me. How I've wronged her.' Tears of shame filled James' eyes. 'That I had so little faith in her. What has she thought of me all these years?'

'You've wronged her deeply,' Tom said, 'and there's no way on God's earth that you can put it right, though you must somehow let her know just how sorry you are. It explains such a lot.' He added, almost to himself.

Annie looked at James as he sat like a broken figure, the scar on his forehead livid against his drained face and tousled hair.

'I'm afraid Pa's right James, things can never be the same again. What's done can't be undone. Her hurt must have been terrible to bear, especially after all she had been through.'

'Don't Ma,' James drew a shuddering breath, 'I know it can never be undone. But there's something I intend to do for her,' he said.

'The legendary horse in Picardie, you told us about?' Tom met James' eyes.

James nodded, 'How will I find a horse in Hertfordshire Pa?'

⚘ ⚘ ⚘

Under the watchful gaze of Gerard O'Malley from his portrait, Tom and James worked in John's study well into the night, reading through files and paperwork, leafing through books on fox hunting, on hunts throughout the country and notable characters connected with them.

'I remember hearing of changes to the Hertfordshire Hunt,' Tom said. 'Originally, it was the famous Hatfield Hunt which we've seen in a couple of these books, that was before my time, but I've heard John speak of his parents connection with them, providing them with horses. Sold them to hunts all over the country as John did in his turn. There's bound to be something in the records but it would take us forever to go through the old files, though we may end up having to.'

He pulled a large red book down from the bookshelf. '*Fox Hunting from Shire to Shire*. When was this published?' He adjusted his glasses and opened the book, turning over a colour plate protected by tissue paper. 'Here we are, 1912, I doubt we'll find anything more recent, taking the war into account that is.' Tom traced down the index with his finger. 'Page 124, Mr. G. Smith-Bosanquet's Hertfordshire pack. I think is what we've been looking for.' He skimmed the pages before saying with satisfaction, 'Broxbornebury Park, Hertfordshire.'

Tom put unheaded writing paper in front of James, 'Write to the hunt and say that you are trying to trace someone you knew in the war, a Captain Thorpe. If he's a horseman, he'll hunt and be known to them. We'll put a stamped return envelope in with the letter for his reply.'

James began to write.

'If we get no reply James, go down there and pursue it. I know that's what John would have done.' He looked up to the mantlepiece at a photograph of John leading Elizabeth on her first pony, 'Elizabeth must know nothing at this stage. I don't want her hopes raised, we've had enough of that with the auctions we've been attending recently.'

❧ ❧ ❧

Elizabeth sat with her aunt at the back of the village church at the funeral of Robert Oakley. Ralph Oakley had made known his wish that she attend. Her mind wandered back to the previous week and the fateful day when Robert had died.

Over and over in her mind she saw the medallion of St. James around James' neck as she experienced again the thunderous shock that it had given her. Then the unbelievable disclosure which had followed. Again, she felt the blood drain from her face as the harrowing truth continued to haunt her. James had believed she had been capable of betraying him, he had taken the word of a man he hated against his belief in her. All these years he had smouldered with his loathing of her. She stared down at the ancient flag stones, how could he have believed this of her, how could he?

Elizabeth knew that her abhorrence of Robert Oakley had died with him. Her emotions towards James however, had flared into incredulity, anger and a hurt so deep that it caused her physical pain.

'Are you alright Elizabeth?' Aunt Martha whispered.

'Yes,' Elizabeth raised her eyes to the frieze around the ceiling of the pre-reformation church, reading the familiar Latin words of the *Credo* which had escaped the despoilers. *Credo*, belief, how little of this James could have had in her, she who had loved him with all her heart.

Following the internment in the family vault, Mrs. Oakley sought out Elizabeth and her aunt and embraced them warmly.

'Elizabeth, Martha, how good of you to come.' She wiped her eyes under her veil, 'Such a sad day.' She took Elizabeth's arm,

'You'll come to the hall? Ralph's expecting to see you there.'

The interior of the hall was swathed in black crepe, curtains and blinds were drawn almost together, emitting only the minimum amount of light. As the day was so cold, with the threat of snow, hot mulled wine was being served in the vestibule as the mourners entered the house. In the pargeted room the funeral meats were spread out on black crepe cloths, the sombre effect broken only by arrangements of white napkins set beside pale plates and silver cutlery.

Elizabeth went over to the Browns, grieving for them that they had not been able to have a funeral for their beloved Saxon, buried in a foreign field. Elizabeth noticed that Edward Brown, their elder son, who was on leave, spent most of the time in the company of Sarah Oakley and it was evident to her that their romance had flourished during their correspondence throughout the war. Elizabeth hoped that they would find happiness together, both having lost brothers. She couldn't help but compare those brothers...

The Burdettes were with the squire, Charles Burdette seated by Ralph and talking earnestly to him. Elizabeth had been pleasantly surprised by the progress the squire had made since she had last seen him, wheelchair bound maybe, but having regained his power of speech and some of his movement on the affected side. As soon as she saw Charles Burdette move on, she crossed the room and knelt by the wheelchair, taking Ralph's hand.

'Elizabeth my dear.' Ralph kissed her cheek, 'Still friends eh, after what my son took from you?'

'Don't worry about any of that today, master.'

'Still master eh? We'll hunt again together yet Elizabeth, show 'em what we're made of.'

'I would very much like to think so.'

'Look forward to it. What with my stroke and the war, the retired huntsman and kennel man have been hunting my hounds. They bring me accounts of the day, keep me up to date.'

She nodded, then put her other hand over his, 'I'm so sorry about your loss.'

'Aye, it's a terrible thing when a man loses his heir, name an' all.' His rheumy eyes filled up. He kept his hand in hers, 'Need to see you when everyone leaves, don't you leave will you?'

'Not if you don't want me to.'

Elizabeth was aware that Victoria was standing behind her. She gently replaced the squire's hand and turned to embrace the girl, 'I'm sorry Victoria.'

'Oh Elizabeth, he was so sweet to me. We've corresponded right through the war as you know. Can you believe that fate could be so awful after all Wobert's been through, that he would die of this terrible influenza?' She began to cry and Elizabeth put her arm around her and endeavoured to comfort her.

Eventually the mourners left. The Oakley family, their retainers and Elizabeth and her aunt were ushered into the library where the squire insisted Elizabeth remain by his side. At Ralph's large, leather topped desk, four men were seated facing the occupants of the room. Elizabeth assumed they were the Oakley family solicitors. The two men on the left she didn't know, the third to her surprise was Mr. Neeson, her solicitor, evidently also retained by the Oakleys. She glanced at the fourth man, it was Mr. Snide, Robert's solicitor. Elizabeth's mouth went dry as she recalled the one and only occasion she had seen this man previously, the terrible day when he had told her that Robert Oakley now owned her home. He caught her looking at him and she averted her eyes as she rose to leave.

Ralph caught her arm, 'Elizabeth no, bear with me.'

Elizabeth remained standing, she could feel that people were beginning to look at her.

Aunt Martha rushed to her side, 'What is it darling? Are you ill?'

Ralph still held her arm, 'Please Elizabeth, stay.'

She looked into his eyes, remembering that he had shown her nothing but kindness all of her life.

'Sit down again by me m'dear.'

Reluctantly, Elizabeth did as she was asked. Mr. Snide began reading Robert's will. The bulk of his interests were left to his parents with a generous gift for each of his sisters. He had left a modest sum for the servants who had been with the family since his childhood and the same for his soldier servant Smith. His personal effects had been distributed amongst his friends. Elizabeth did not feature amongst any of it. Then Sarah, Hannah and the servants were asked to leave the library.

Ralph's solicitor cleared his throat, 'I have been given instructions by Squire Oakley,' he began, opening a file and placing it in front of him, 'of an unusual nature. As you have already heard, Captain Oakley left the bulk of his estate to his parents. Included in that estate is the property formerly known as the O'Malley Stud Farm which Captain Oakley,' here he coughed a couple of times, 'acquired by means of a card game. It is the express wish of Squire and Mrs. Oakley to return the said property in its entirety to Miss Elizabeth O'Malley Sullivan.'

Elizabeth gasped with disbelief, she stared at Ralph open mouthed.

He nodded to her confidently, 'Fair dues Elizabeth, fair dues.'

She covered her mouth with her hand, then reached into her bag for a handkerchief to staunch the tears which were stinging her eyes.

'Miss O'Malley Sullivan's solicitor, Mr. Neeson is here today to commence the transaction with Mr. Snide. All should be completed within one month.' He looked to Snide, who glared at him.

Elizabeth was in a daze. She remembered her aunt and Lenora hugging her and Mr. Neeson and Ralph's solicitor shaking her hand and then being left alone in the library with Ralph and kneeling by his chair. She reached for his hand as she thanked him and he patted her back, clumsily.

'Keep it close to the chest for the month Elizabeth and then I hope you'll move back home. Be neighbours again eh? Like the old days.'

※ ※ ※

James' letter was answered by one of the hunt servants.

'Yes, he knew Captain Thorpe well, hunted regularly before the war. Of course any friend of his would be aware of the terrible injuries he had sustained. Bound to appreciate contact from a friend he'd made in the war. Still lived at the same place, Westwood Hall, Westwood, near Stanstead Abbots.'

'That's it,' Tom said with satisfaction. 'Do you want me to go with you? I mean, it's your show.'

'I'd appreciate it if you did Pa, it's good of you.'

'That's settled then, see the horse somehow and if by a miracle it is Rua, then we shall know him alright.' He looked directly at James, 'I don't think we'll be very welcome, but never the less, we must go. Take a pony and trap to the station tomorrow and book our tickets.'

Four days later, Tom and James were walking along what seemed to them an endless country road. Tufts of faded grass grew in the middle of it and they had seen no one since asking directions at the station. The day was bitingly cold and an east wind cut through them, the bare hedges each side of the road affording little or no protection. James was in uniform and had been grateful for the thick army greatcoat over his tunic, but now he felt he was hauling it along as his leg grew more and more painful. How long, he thought, aware of sweat breaking out on his top lip, would his damned leg give him this much gyp? He cast a sidelong glance at Tom, who was battling along gamely, giving no indication that he had noticed James' stride becoming more and more uneven.

Eventually, they passed a few houses and after rounding a bend, on a hill to their right, a large house came into view of four square Palladian architecture. As they drew nearer, they could see outbuildings and stables to the south of it, in the same inimitable style: Westwood Hall, as described by the person who had given them directions.

James slowed down, feeling his stomach turn over. He glanced at Tom and pulled a face.

Tom returned the grimace but didn't slacken his pace, 'Come on James, no time now for faint heart, just think of the trouble you've gone to already to get this far.'

James nodded, reassured by Tom's words which reminded him momentarily of his childhood and the self confidence which Tom had always given him.

An elderly manservant opened the door, a wisp of his white hair raised by the wind as he looked at them enquiringly.

'Would it be possible to see Captain Thorpe?' James began.

'Is he expecting you?'

'Probably not,' James said. 'But we've travelled a long way hoping to see him.'

The man ran his fingers through his hair as the wind continued to blow it about. 'Perhaps you'd better come inside,' he said.

Tom and James did as he asked, accepting hard chairs next to the door in a large circular entrance hall where a log fire was reflected in the marble floor.

'If you wait here, I'll enquire if Captain Thorpe is at home.'

It was some time before the man returned. 'The Captain is not at home,' he informed them as he began to unfasten the door.

James felt dismay born of bitter disappointment wash through him. He rose and faced the man, 'Please go back to him and tell him we've called about a horse. I've just returned from France. I have a note for him from Jacques Vautrin. It's a matter of importance.'

The servant demurred for a moment and as he turned from them a voice from an open door opposite, echoed through the hall.

'Alright Hodgkins, show them into the library.'

Tom and James saw a man held up by crutches struggling to manoeuvre himself across the floor. He had a horrific scar the length of his forehead and his right leg was bound in bandages from top to bottom. His progress was slow and James recalled hearing Monique speak of a serious chest injury.

Once in the library, perfunctory introductions were made and it was apparent that Captain Thorpe was not only ill at ease but was suppressing other emotions, not least, annoyance.

'Now, what's all this about?' He looked directly at James.

'We're sorry to disturb you sir, all we ask is to see the horse you recently had brought over from France.'

'Horse from France?' Captain Thorpe laughed dryly, 'I know nothing of a horse from France. Are you talking about the recent auctions of army surplus horses?'

'No, sir, I'm talking about this horse.' From his pocket James pulled out the short note from Jacques and passed it over. James knew the words by heart as he watched the man read.

'Mon Capitan, The bearer of this note, James Gretton, says he was at the commandeering of a horse he believes to be *le Rouge*. He has been persistent in harassing myself and Henri. I believe him to be totally trustworthy and sincere, otherwise neither Henri, Monique or myself would have taken him into our confidence. Whether or not *le Rouge* is the horse in question we all feel that once he has seen it he will be satisfied. We send our regards, Jacques Vautrin.'

'Who else knows of this?'

'No one, except of course, my father here.'

'How have you come to hear of this, possibly imaginary horse?'

'I heard its story told whilst I was in a hospital near St. Emilie. It had been generally supposed that the horse died of its injuries.'

'And?'

'After the soldier had finished telling the story and everyone had lost interest, he added that the horse was a red stallion.'

Captain Thorpe was quiet for a moment and then asked, 'Have you any intention of taking this ridiculous story to the authorities?'

James stared at him, indignation evident in his eyes, 'I would never do such a thing.'

His words hung in the silence which followed and then Tom spoke.

'Captain you have our word that this whole business is in complete confidence, we are horsemen, we share a mutual bond. We know the horse my son traced in France is now here, all we ask is that you allow us to see it. Whether or not it is Rua, it must be an incredible animal. You have risked much for its survival and we respect that.'

'Rua?'

'O'Malley Ri Rua.'

'O'Malley?' Captain Thorpe was perceptively startled. 'O'Malley horses have always been highly coveted around here. What exactly is your interest in an O'Malley horse?'

Tom answered him, 'I was stud groom to the late John O'Malley Sullivan, he was my employer and best friend. I manage what's left of the business now for his daughter. My son grew up at the stud, he was, along with Miss O'Malley at the birth of Rua. They both worked with him and later saw him commandeered.'

Captain Thorpe frowned, 'They commandeered horses from such a stud?'

'They plundered it.'

❦ ❦ ❦

A young man was summoned and introduced as Captain Thorpe's soldier servant Bridges, who helped his officer into a wheelchair and led Tom and James out of the house, across an area of cobblestones and through the Doric archway of an imposing stable block. They crossed the yard and passed through a second arch into a smaller yard, tucked away, with a few stables down one side of it. A grassed area on the open side led onto a high railed paddock of about, James estimated, two acres.

James knew they were near the horse, he felt his mouth go dry and his legs become weak. He stood for a moment and then whistled, once, long and low. He knew by the horse's response that it was Rua even before he saw him. Two whinnies were followed by his head over a stable door. James went to him, rubbing his face on that of the horse whilst talking in a quiet voice. The horse nickered and mumbled his recognition. Those watching were visibly moved.

'Lead him out Bridges, would you?' Captain Thorpe asked, nodding as the man hesitated for a moment.

Bridges disappeared into what James supposed was a tack room, emerging with a strong headstall, a stallion's headstall.

James followed him into the loose box, watching the horse's impeccable manners as the headstall was fitted, then followed them out as Bridges led Rua around the grass. As the man turned to lead him the opposite way round, James saw the massive scar on the animal's shoulder, the skin around bare of hair and if the horse dropped at all on its near side, James decided it was minimal. The wound had been as Jacques described it.

Bridges brought the horse up to the group, Rua seemed so much bigger to James, who was aware that like himself the horse had grown and matured during the years of war.

Captain Thorpe reached out and fondled the red muzzle, 'Well Gretton, there's no doubt, I suppose?'

'No sir, it's Rua.'

'Glad you've seen him,' he saw James look at Tom. 'No, I mean it, put your minds at rest and you've given me a name for him.'

Back at the house, James found that Captain Thorpe's attitude had mellowed somewhat. He offered them tea, apologising for the absence of his wife and seated in front of a fire in the library, told them of his hopes.

'Don't know how long it will be before I'll ride again. What a ride *le Rouge* was, but then you know all about that. I'm considering breeding horses, the idea has been growing in my head since my second set of injuries.' He laughed without humour. 'Had to go back for another innings, wasn't up to it, but neither were thousands of others, just had to get on with it didn't we Gretton?'

James nodded, his head teeming with thoughts, memories, and the overwhelming magnitude of actually having found Rua.

Captain Thorpe looked hard at him and said quietly, 'Make no mistake, I shall never give him up. I owe my life to him, he's everything to me.'

Tom turned to him, 'We can understand that, but may we ask another favour of you.'

The Captain looked sceptical as Tom continued, 'Would you permit us to bring Miss O'Malley to see him?'

XXVII

Tom and James returned home late evening. Annie was over-whelmed by their news. Although she had commended their efforts, she had been unable to make herself believe that it would be possible to trace an O'Malley horse, least of all the stallion which had meant so much to them all.

James had taken the dogs for their run and Tom and Annie were talking, whilst waiting for him to return for supper.

'The job now then, is to break the news to Elizabeth,' Annie said, pouring Tom a tankard of cider. She glanced sideways at him, 'Do you really think it's wise Tom? I can't help but wonder if it would be best to let sleeping dogs lie.'

Tom stared at her in disbelief, 'What are you thinking of Annie? How we have scoured the army auctions these past weeks and after all James has done to trace this horse. I think it will be the making of her, just to know that Rua has survived and has a home in a million.'

'Perhaps I understand Elizabeth a bit better than you do,' Annie said quietly. 'A home in a million to her, will be with her. She'll want to take him up to Derbyshire where she's considering having the farm-house restored and rebuilding the business when she comes of age.'

'How do you know this?' Tom asked incredulously.

'Because Elizabeth mentioned it in the letter she left with me the day she came over, she didn't see the point of posting it when she was seeing us. She said she wanted to talk to us, but after all that hap-pened... I put it in my pocket and I've only just read it.'

'For God's sake, Annie.'

'I'm sorry Tom, it's just that I've been worried sick about every-thing.'

'What will she think of us, not mentioning it? This explains what she meant when she called in the day of Captain Oakley's funeral. She said she had some incredible news for us in a month, remember?'

'That will be it then, moving to Gatthorpe. Though I don't know whether I'd call it incredible news.' Annie said dubiously.

'Would Martha move with her?'

'No, Elizabeth says not, she's upset about that, but who can blame Martha? She's not an O'Malley after all. I suppose she'd stay whilst Elizabeth settles, but it's all in the air at the moment.'

'Circumstances have changed since she wrote that letter Annie. This place will be a much safer tenancy now, under the squire. Elizabeth's bound to know that.' Annie nodded in agreement.

Tom stared into the fire and took a pull at his cider. 'Knowing now what happened between James and Elizabeth has put us in a difficult situation.'

Annie sat down beside him, 'You've done well by Elizabeth as John trusted you would, but she's almost twenty one now and our first loyalty has to be to James, you've said so yourself.' She put her hand on his arm as he began to interrupt her, 'He needs us more than you think, he's at rock bottom Tom.'

'Aye, do you think I don't know that Annie.'

James could be heard outside whistling to the dogs. Annie got up and crossed to the range, taking out a large meat and potato pie which she placed on the table.

'He wants me to be the one to tell her about the horse and take her to see him.' Tom told her.

Annie was setting out plates, 'Perhaps Martha's brother-in-law will offer to take her, he's trailed around the auctions with her.'

'Wouldn't be the same, he seems a grand chap and he's been very good to Elizabeth, but he's no horseman.'

'And it takes a horseman to accompany her to Hertfordshire does it?'

'Indeed it does.'

❧ ❧ ❧

Martha looked up from her breakfast, seeing Elizabeth with a letter from Tom in her hand. To her concern, Elizabeth's eyes were filled with tears.

'Whatever is it, please God not more bad news?'

'Aunt, it's the best of news. Tom has found one of my horses.'

'Not really?'

Elizabeth read on, 'It seems that James traced it in France and then to England, where Tom discovered where it had been taken to.'

She was silent as she continued to read, 'Aunt, it's Rua...' She let the letter fall as she put her elbows on the table and covered her face with her hands. Martha waited for a while, then went to her and put her arm across the girl's shoulders.

Elizabeth looked up at her aunt, her face tear stained and radiant, 'They've actually seen him.'

'I'm so happy for you my dear, I must be honest, I didn't think there was the slightest chance of you ever seeing any of them again.' She picked up the letter and handed it back to Elizabeth.

Elizabeth wiped her eyes and resumed reading, turning the page, 'The person who brought him from France has agreed to me seeing him. Tom has asked if we can go next week, possible Wednesday. He's waiting now for a reply. He finishes by saying that we keep this to ourselves. Of course we shall. I shall hug it to me. Just over a week, all being well. How can I wait that long?'

'Darling, be patient. You've waited for four years.'

Elizabeth was not patient, she wrote back to Tom instantly and then threw herself into every time consuming activity that she could think of in an effort to speed up the time. She turned her aunt's attic inside out, a job which Martha had been putting off for years, worked alongside the gardener, who helped Martha out occasionally, digging out and pruning back many of the shrubs which Martha had also been putting off, and on the days when she was on duty at Collingswell Hall, worked in a frenzy which did not enhance her popularity with either the staff or the other volunteers.

She scanned the post each morning and some days later was

rewarded by another letter from Tom.

'It is to be Wednesday,' she read. 'We shall travel to Hertfordshire together and see my horse.'

'Elizabeth, you must remember that he's not your horse now. If the person who is responsible for bringing him from France has bought him from the army, then the horse belongs to him.'

'At the moment, yes, I know that. But he'll always be my horse. How could he be any other?'

Martha didn't pursue it. She knew Tom well enough to accept that he would talk to Elizabeth.

✄ ✄ ✄

Elizabeth clung to her aunt before boarding the train for Nottingham. It was, she felt in some indefinable way, as though both of them were aware that a phase of life was over and that things would not be quite the same again. This portent of destiny linked with great euphoria persisted throughout the journey and lasted until she jumped off the train in Nottingham Midland Station eager to meet Tom.

Tom was not there. James was.

Elizabeth stood motionless on the platform. Her first thought was to get back into the train, get away from him, no matter where.

He walked towards her, 'Elizabeth.'

Elizabeth today is it? she thought as she lifted her chin and faced him.

'Where's Tom?'

'He's ill.'

Her heart sank, 'Not the 'flu, please tell me it's not the 'flu?'

'We don't know what it is, he took ill yesterday and by this morning he was no better. Ma made him go back to bed and she's going to send for Doctor Morley.'

'Dear God, I've never known Tom go to bed in the daytime. We mustn't think of going.'

'He insisted. In fact when I told him I'd meet you and tell you it was off, he began to get very upset. Ma thought it best we go. That's what he wants.'

Elizabeth felt numb, much as she craved to see Rua, she couldn't bear Tom being ill. She bit her lip. 'I still think we shouldn't go.'

'It's up to you, I've told you what he wants us to do.'

'What do you really think?' Elizabeth felt herself blushing, what she had just said reminded her of the old days and the absolute trust she'd had in him.

'I prefer to do as Pa wishes.'

Elizabeth nodded slowly, 'What time does the train leave?'

'We've half an hour to get to Victoria Station. Joe's waiting outside with the trap.'

If Elizabeth considered the journey across town to be an embarrassment, she had not then experienced the journey to Hertfordshire. The atmosphere between them was like a wall.

Where normally she would have resented sharing a carriage with strangers, on this occasion she was almost grateful for their presence. When she had felt she was not overheard and for the minutes when the carriage had emptied at different stations, she had several times endeavoured to find out how he had traced Rua in France, but he was totally unforthcoming and finally she gave up. She found, that like James, she too was purposely avoiding any eye contact. They were, she felt, like strangers who had little or nothing in common. It was as though he had pulled down shutters, when there was so much she desperately wanted to know.

How she wished that Tom was there, but he would tell her everything when she saw him. A chill stole through her, what if anything happened to Tom? She couldn't bear it, especially now when she had less than two weeks before telling him and Annie that the stud had been restored to her. Surely fate couldn't be so cruel? But it could, as she knew only too well. She examined her feelings as she stared out of the carriage window. The tremendous anticipation of seeing Rua was still as potent, despite her anxiety for Tom, but James' distant attitude following his awareness of the truth between them was anathema to her. The journey seemed interminable, despite the change of trains at Grantham.

Captain Thorpe had sent transport to the station in the form of a Bentley motor car which made the journey to Westwood more comfortable for James, although he would sooner have died than admitted it. He looked out of the car's windows at the lanes along which he and Tom had walked less than two weeks before. He felt again their shared hope of seeing Rua once more and their immeasurable joy in doing so. He understood how Elizabeth would be feeling, although she appeared outwardly calm, detached from him. What could he expect? God, how could he have been so wrong, so certain of her betrayal. He tried to imagine what it would have been like for her, coming home after her illness, her first thought to find him.

Ma had told him how frail she had been and how she had collapsed when she had learned he had left. Then her attempt to contact him by the tentative letter she had sent him, her only letter and he had destroyed it. He felt himself writhe, how she must hate him and he had only himself to blame. No, he thought, not only himself, that bastard Robert Oakley, he'd done nothing but harm to Elizabeth and she hadn't seen it until it was too late. Too late. Even in death, Robert Oakley had won.

The car drew onto the gravel. This time Captain Thorpe himself opened the door to them. James introduced them.

Captain Thorpe took Elizabeth hand, 'It's a great pleasure for me to meet an O'Malley, the name has always carried a lot of clout with the Hertfordshire Hunt...' He stared at her, 'Though I must confess I was expecting an elderly hunting type.'

Elizabeth smiled, 'Hunting type maybe, elderly, not quite yet.'

'May I offer you some refreshment after your journey?'

'No, really, thank you.'

'You're anxious to see the horse?'

'I am, even to the point of rudeness.'

He nodded his understanding and summoned Bridges.

Elizabeth felt as though she was wading through treacle, her legs weighed her down and she felt almost incapable of following Captain Thorpe and Bridges across the large yard to the smaller one.

James behind her, was aware of her hesitant step, which the tilt of her head sought to deny. As they passed through the second arch, he gave the long, low whistle, then drew alongside her, watching her as they were greeted by two whinnies and then the horse looked out over the half door.

'Rua,' Elizabeth's voice was barely a whisper. She went to him and did exactly as James had done, she lay her face against his and listened to his sounds of recognition. None of the men moved, all three were transfixed, watching the beautiful dark haired girl and the red stallion.

For James, it was the picture which had carried him through war.

❧ ❧ ❧

Following lunch at the insistence of his wife, Captain Thorpe asked Elizabeth, 'Did you used to ride him?'

She looked at James, 'I, we, broke him in, schooled him. Yes, I rode him all the time. Papa wasn't overkeen on riding an entire so much, but he was sheer joy to ride, as you must have found.'

Captain Thorpe nodded, 'How would you feel about riding him today?'

'Tom said he'd been injured.'

'That was two years ago, it was touch and go with him for some time, but he's made a good recovery. He owes his life to some people in France. He's fine, ridden with care.'

'I have no riding clothes with me.'

'My sister has plenty, you're about her size. What do you think?'

Elizabeth's eyes shone, 'I think yes, definitely yes,' she said.

'Do you ride side saddle or astride?'

'Both. The horse is used to both, but I prefer to ride him astride, I'm in closer contact with him.'

❧ ❧ ❧

Bridges had Rua saddled up and was leading him around the railed off paddock when Elizabeth, Captain Thorpe and James returned to the stables. Elizabeth was kitted out in breeches, boots and a jacket which were not too bad a fit. Her heart was thumping and she took deep breaths to enable herself to be a calming influence on Rua. James followed her into the paddock. He went up to the horse, stroked its neck and automatically adjusted the stirrup leathers to her length, then cupped his hands to give her a leg up. Just as automatically Elizabeth put her knee into his hands as he threw her lightly up onto the horse.

She settled herself into the saddle, gathered up the reins and felt Rue's sides with her calves. His head was up and his ears pricked, his red mane fluttered in the winter breeze. She walked him around the perimeter and then put him into a trot, perfectly balanced and controlled. As she rode across the far side of the paddock, she urged the horse into an extended trot. James heard Captain Thorpe catch his breath as he watched the powerful floating action which Elizabeth and himself had taught the stallion over four years before.

Elizabeth rejoiced in the familiar warmth of the horse against her legs as he picked up her aids and she was exquisitely aware of the long remembered evocative smell of him which took her back to days full of horses, security and young love.

Seeing them together, a thought revolved around and around Captain Thorpe's head like a mantra. He tried to dismiss it, almost angrily, but it would not leave him. He was home, the horse was not.

✄ ✄ ✄

James hurriedly swallowed a cup of tea in the library and then excused himself, to return to the horse. Elizabeth would like to have done the same, but as well as feeling it would be churlish, she knew that it would defeat James' objective, he wished to be relieved of her presence.

'What breeding stock do you have now Miss O'Malley?' Captain Thorpe enquired when James had left.

'There are mares at the Derbyshire holding who are more than overdue for serving and mares and young stock in Ireland.' She smiled, 'Thanks to the vigilance of my relatives in Ireland, there's a good possibility of recovering many of our bloodlines. We sent what we could over there following the commandeering whilst we were able to and kept only very young stock here.'

'It must have been hell for you.'

'It was.'

'Will you have any mares to sell?'

'Why do you ask?'

'I thought Mr. Sharkey and Gretton would have told you, I hope to breed horses myself.'

'In that case you could rely on mares from us, I could never repay what you've done for Rua.'

Captain Thorpe looked at his leg, 'I don't know when or if I'll be much good riding again and whilst I don't expect any return from *le Rouge*, sorry, Rua, I'm now convinced that his true role will be at stud.'

'Oh absolutely, why as soon as he was born, James and I began to make plans for his future.'

There was an uncomfortable silence before Captain Thorpe spoke again, 'I made it perfectly clear to Mr. Sharkey and Gretton, that I have no intention of parting with the horse. Did they not inform you of this Miss O'Malley?'

Elizabeth felt torn between an understanding of the badly injured man and her own hopes of Rua being restored to her. She said diplomatically, 'Unfortunately I haven't had the opportunity of speaking to Mr. Sharkey regarding his visit here. He wrote to me of course.' Then added by way of explanation, 'Mr. Sharkey and his wife still live at the stud premises, but I've spent almost the last four years with my aunt in Lincoln.'

'He seems to have your interests very much at heart, as does his son. I must say I can't help but admire Gretton for his dogged perseverance in tracing the horse.'

Elizabeth's face softened, 'We grew up together. James was my best friend.'

'Was?'

'It's all a long story captain, like so many people at this time, our lives have been turned upside down. Now if you'll permit me, I'll go and see Rua again before we leave.'

❧ ❧ ❧

Elizabeth and James had to rush to catch the train. They stood some distance from each other, in the corridor to recover. James glanced at her, bewitched by her flushed face and dark lashed eyes.

'What is it?' she asked raising her chin and for the first time that day, their eyes met.

'Nothing.'

'James, I so much want you to tell me about your search for Rua. Captain Thorpe mentioned it, but I could only listen to what he volunteered.' She stared down at the floor. 'To be honest, I didn't want him to discover that I know so little of your quest. I felt it would seem odd to him.'

James looked at her hesitantly.

'Please James, surely you know me well enough to understand how desperately I want to hear the story from you?'

He looked into her eyes, still hesitant, feeling that his search for Rua seemed so long ago. It had been done in the days when he had thought more of finding the horse than any acknowledged thought of her. Now his bitterness and disillusionment had been turned upside down, she had done him no wrong, perhaps that was why fate had been kind to her for once in the finding of Rua. For all the turmoil in his mind, he knew he owed her the facts and so began to relate them to her from when he had first heard the story of the horse. When he told her how Rua had carried his rider to safety, both of them gravely wounded, she wept.

He was painfully aware that Elizabeth watched his face the whole time, every feature, every expression and listened intently to his every word. He brought her up to date, to the present day when she had seen and ridden the horse, then looked away from her, his eyes giving nothing away.

'James.'

Reluctantly, he turned back to her.

'Thank you,' she said.

When they boarded the next train, James hung back by the door. 'Elizabeth, could we stay near the door, it's impossible to talk in the carriages.'

They faced each other and Elizabeth felt intensely conscious of his closeness, just inches from her. She sensed that he was equally ill at ease, she felt his eyes upon her and looked at him questioningly.

After a while, he spoke, 'This may be my last and only opportunity of speaking to you about what's happened between us.'

She turned her face to the window. Through the dark reflection she saw him close his eyes as he rubbed a hand across his forehead. The gesture of hopelessness went through her and she turned back to him.

'Please Elizabeth, it has to be talked about, for the sake of what we had if nothing else. God knows it's hard enough for me to face you after I learned the truth. I've known all day what I wanted to say, but I didn't know where to start. It has to be said.'

Elizabeth looked directly at him, his eyes she noticed were as she had once seen them in a hayfield an eternity ago, large black pupils surrounded by pure grey. He pushed his fingers through his hair in the way she long remembered.

'You must understand and always know, that I feel nothing for myself but loathing, I don't believe that will ever change. No matter how much you despise me, I despise myself a thousand times more. I shall have to live my life with the knowledge of what I, who... God forgive me, loved you so much, did to you, through no fault of yours.'

He covered his face with his hands as he strove to bring himself under control. 'Our paths won't cross again, I promise you. I'm moving out as soon as Pa's better. I know Ma told you I have a place. You'll not be troubled by my presence again. To say that I'm sorry just isn't enough. I should never, ever have believed anything bad about you. You kept faith Beth, I did not.'

His voice was low and husky with emotion, his eyes were full of pain and to her distress were brimming with tears. She realised that in all her life she had never seen him cry, though he had comforted her hundreds of times. How could she live her life never seeing him again as he had promised? How could she face the future without him? She felt a churning mix of emotions, gratitude for his tenacity in tracing Rua, grief for what he had so cruelly and unexpectedly been led to believe, and horror at his wretched degradation at the hands of Robert Oakley.

She couldn't bear to see him so distressed, she felt his pain tearing into her as she was overcome by compassion for his suffering, which like her own had been so needless, so cruel. Standing close to him she felt magnetised by his proximity, filled with an overwhelming longing to lay her head on his chest against the reefer jacket he was wearing, to feel his lips on the top of her head and for him to lift her chin with his hand and kiss her mouth like he used to. She swayed towards him and he caught her arms to steady her, then she felt him release his grip, he was letting her go. But he didn't, he began to put his arms about her, tentatively.

'Hold me James, hold me tight.'

He took her into his arms and she felt him kiss the top of her head and then he put his hand under her chin and raised her face as he lowered his head and kissed her mouth and she tasted the salt of his tears.

※ ※ ※

At Nottingham Victoria Station, Joe Bingley was already waiting with the trap. James and Elizabeth rushed to him.

Joe touched his cap, 'Evening Miss Elizabeth, James.'

'How is he Joe, how's Pa?'

His face was solemn and Elizabeth felt her face blanch as they waited for his reply.

'He's about the same, yet he flatly refuses to have Doctor Morley sent for.'

'We'll see about that when I get home. Elizabeth's coming back with me, we're worried sick about him.' James sorted some change for Elizabeth and waited whilst she left a message for her aunt with Wilfred on his recently installed telephone. She explained that Tom was ill and she was going to Oakley to see him.

⚜ ⚜ ⚜

Annie heard the pony and trap pull into the yard, 'He's here, quick get up to bed.'

Tom, looking his usual robust self, took his feet out of the hearth and disappeared through the stairfoot door. After Joe had reassured James that he needed no help with the pony, James took Elizabeth's hand and led her towards the cottage. When the sound of the pony's hooves had gone, they put their arms around each other and made for the door.

Tom watching from a darkened upstairs window, was content.

EPILOGUE

In April, 1926, a memorial was unveiled in London, at the Church of St. Judes-on-the-hill, Hampstead Garden Suburb, inscribed with the following words:

> *'In grateful memory of the Empire horses, some 375,000, who fell in the Great War 1914-18. Most obediently and often most painfully they died, faithful unto death. Not one is forgotten before God.'*

James and Elizabeth O'Malley Gretton were present.

ACKNOWLEDGMENTS

I would like to offer my sincere thanks to everyone who has helped with the research and writing of this book, including reference books and organisations as follows:

Historical Records of the South Nottinghamshire Yeomanry Hussars 1794-1924 by the late George Fellows, Major, South Notts. Yeomanry Cavalry and the late Benson Freeman OBE, Fellow of the Royal Hist. Soc., Engineer Commander, Royal Navy (retired);

The Royal British Legion; Staff of Nottingham City Libraries; *Nottingham Evening Post* archives; Veterans of the Great War; Florence Wilson, my mother, for her childhood memories of the commandeering of horses and of Armistice Day; *Fox Hunting from Shire to Shire* by Cuthbert Bradley, 1912; the late Anne Wilson MFH Barlow Hunt; Anne Bower; Dudley Fowkes, Midland Railway Trust; Maryck Holloway for French translations; Dawn Robertson and staff at Hayloft Publishing, and all those who have, in their different ways, supported and encouraged this work - many thanks to all.

Jennifer Appleyard, 2012

THE AUTHOR

Jennifer Appleyard lives in a small village west of Nottingham with her husband David. They have two daughters and eight grand children who spend school holidays with them, riding and helping at shows with their rare breed White Park cattle.

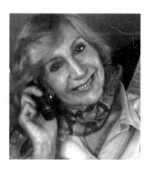

In the 1970s Jennifer first wrote the story of Elizabeth and James, inspired by her love of horses and her family's experiences during the Great War. In 2001 during the foot and mouth epidemic when activities were curtailed and the constant fear of the disease hung over them, she began to write again in earnest and, amongst other work, rewrote this story. She is currently working on a sequel.

Photo: John Daniels